CLOSE YOUR EYES . . .
Lose Weight

Also by Grace Smith

Close Your Eyes, Get Free (2017)

CLOSE YOUR EYES . . .
Lose Weight

Reprogram Your Subconscious Mind
in Twelve Weeks to Eat Healthy,
Feel Great, and Love Your Body with the
Groundbreaking Power of Hypnosis

Grace Smith

BenBella Books, Inc.
Dallas, TX

BenBella Books, Inc.
10440 N. Central Expressway, Suite 800
Dallas, TX 75231
www.benbellabooks.com
Send feedback to feedback@benbellabooks.com

BenBella is a federally registered trademark.

Printed in the United States of America
10 9 8 7 6 5 4 3 2 1

Library of Congress Cataloging-in-Publication is available upon request.
ISBN 9781950665020 (print)
ISBN 9781950665198 (electronic)

Copyediting by Miki Alexandra Caputo
Proofreading by Michael Fedison and Beth M. Custer
Text design and composition by Aaron Edmiston
Cover design by Emily Weigel
Printed by Versa Press

Distributed to the trade by Two Rivers Distribution, an Ingram brand
www.tworiversdistribution.com

Special discounts for bulk sales are available.
Please contact bulkorders@benbellabooks.com.

For my clients,
whose transformations inspire me to no end.

Your journey extends beyond the book!

Visit www.CloseYourEyesLoseWeight.com to access free bonus resources, including more than a dozen hypnosis audio recordings for weight loss.

Contents

PREFACE:

. . . .

Why Hypnosis Will Work (When Nothing Else Has)

Weight loss. A multibillion-dollar industry. Day in and day out you're sold solutions. "Quick-fix" diets and supplements. Liquids and powders. Exercise mats and smart watches. Apps and smart monitors. Thigh-gap machines and detox programs. But does the multibillion-dollar weight loss industrial complex want you to lose weight and keep it off? Absolutely not! They make their money if the struggle continues, not if you finally discover a lasting solution. You already know that get-thin-quick diets don't work in the long term. You already know hating your body doesn't cause it to lose weight. And yet, fad diets, self-hatred, negative self-talk, and gimmicky products prevail.

If you feel duped by the weight loss industry, you're not alone.

A body mass index (BMI) of 30 or over is considered obese, but in 2016 the average woman in the United States was 170 pounds and five foot three with a BMI of 29.6; the average man was 197 pounds and five foot seven with a BMI of 29.1.[1] This puts the *average* American on the cusp of obesity.

While BMI, a value derived from the mass and height of a person, isn't necessarily the best or only way to assess health, it can be a useful reference point and a potentially helpful screening tool for overweightness or obesity.

The obesity epidemic is not confined to one country. The World Health Organization has issued the following key facts:

- Worldwide obesity has nearly tripled since 1975.
- In 2016, more than 1.9 billion adults, 18 years and older, were overweight. Of these over 650 million were obese.
- 39% of adults aged 18 years and over were overweight in 2016, and 13% were obese.
- Most of the world's population live in countries where overweight and obesity kill more people than underweight.
- 41 million children under the age of 5 were overweight or obese in 2016.

---

1 Cheryl D. Fryar et al., *Mean Body Weight, Height, Waist Circumference, and Body Mass Index Among Adults: United States, 1999–2000 Through 2015–2016*, National Health Statistics Report no. 122, December 20, 2018, https://cdc.gov/nchs/data/nhsr/nhsr122-508.pdf.

- Over 340 million children and adolescents aged 5–19 were overweight or obese in 2016.
- Obesity is preventable.[2]

How can the average American be nearly obese when there is a multibillion-dollar weight loss industrial complex?

The truth is, the vast majority of the weight loss industry doesn't want you to lose weight, they don't want you to look better, and they don't want you to *feel* better. Not in the long run, anyway. Pushing misery and failure sells far more products than promoting happiness and long-term health does.

Literally thousands of books recommend a diet that "is the only one that works." Every five years two dozen new books crop up telling you why those now outdated diets are toxic and disease causing and why you need this new, equally extreme diet instead. The system is rigged to keep you buying more and more.

But enough cynicism. You're here to change your life, and that requires courage, energy, and a positive outlook! While it's important to know what you're up against, it's far more important to focus on the solution rather than the problem. Rather than tackling the behemoth of contradictory and confusing information that is the "weight loss" field, we're going to link arms together and take the road much, much less traveled.

This book will not tout any particular diet, besides eating real foods that come from the earth and weren't made in a laboratory.

This book will not teach any particular exercise routine outside of simply making it a priority to move your body until it releases endorphins.

---

2 "Obesity and Overweight," World Health Organization, February 16, 2018, www.who.int/news-room/fact-sheets/detail/obesity-and-overweight.

This book will not give you new food recommendations or exercise plans because there is already plenty of good material from doctors, dietitians, and personal trainers (although in the bonus materials available at www.CloseYourEyesLoseWeight.com, I will recommend my favorite experts from these fields, along with a certified nutritionist's suggested meal plan and recipe ideas).

This book is different from other weight loss books out there.

This book was written for your *sub*conscious mind, and that is the precise reason this book will have a tremendously positive impact on your life. The subconscious is "the totality of mental processes of which the individual is not aware."[3] In other words, the subconscious is where the root of your habits, beliefs, and emotional responses lives. It's an important place. The foundations of ALL your habits. ALL your beliefs. And ALL your emotional responses. Yet no one has ever taught you how to access and upgrade this almighty place of importance—until now.

I hope you will find what follows to feel like a breath of fresh air—clean, clear, light, invigorating, energizing. In fact, take a nice, deep letting-go breath now and allow yourself to relax deeper into the realization that you are about to experience something that is likely brand new for you.

Even more important, I know you will find in these pages something we all desire yet is hard to come by—results. Lasting results.

If you want to eat differently, fall in love with your magnificent body, and release emotional weight, then you will have to access your subconscious mind directly to do it. This book teaches you how.

---

3 Dictionary.com, s.v. "subconscious (*n.*)" accessed November 3, 2019, s.v.www. dictionary.com/browse/subconscious.

Allow Me to (Very Briefly) Introduce Myself

I want to share with you the most important highlights of my background so you can have confidence in this book and the results that await you.

In 2010 I was living in the Lower East Side of New York City, working in a corporate job with long hours, big quotas to reach, and crushing stress. My days of partying as a "coping mechanism" were recently behind me and I wanted to quit smoking, but nothing seemed to work. Patches, gum, cold turkey, books on how to quit, I tried them all, but months after setting my first, then second, then third "quit date" I was still a smoker, even though I desperately wanted to stop.

Someone suggested I get hypnotized to quit smoking. It was an interesting idea, but I had massive reservations. Besides conjuring up creepy mind-control images of stage hypnotists, I thought, "I am incapable of relaxing enough to get hypnotized." Still, I had nothing to lose, so I booked a hypnotherapy session.

And it worked.

I had been smoking a pack a day, yet, despite my reservations, I managed to quit in one session even when I didn't believe it would work. Following my first session, I had two more to seal the deal, and after that any lingering cravings were gone, too. Immediately after these hypnotherapy sessions, some questions came to mind: Why is anyone smoking who doesn't want to smoke? Why did I think this would be creepy mind control or clucking chickens when in fact it was one of the most relaxing, reassuring, fascinating experiences I've ever had? Why did I think this wouldn't work when it was the *only* thing that did work . . . and so quickly? What is the subconscious? Why doesn't everyone know what hypnosis *really* is? Why is using hypnosis to access the subconscious so effective at making lasting change? What is going on here?!

To me, the fact that people were suffering needlessly by smoking when they didn't want to smoke was a human rights issue. I had to learn more.

Cut to a number of months later. I'd become a certified hypnotherapist, still working in a corporate job full-time but growing more and more enthralled with my side gig. My clients' results were taking my breath away, but it wasn't until I met Alexandre, Alex for short (whose story I tell in full in chapter one of my book *Close Your Eyes, Get Free*), that I saw what hypnosis could do.

You see, Alex, who had been paralyzed by a stroke for over three months, could not move a muscle on the left side of his body. Forty-five minutes into our very first hypnotherapy session together, Alex **broke through his paralysis** and voluntarily moved his left hand for the first time. Needless to say, neither of our lives have been the same since.

The Wellness Institute has a medical explanation for how it was possible for Alexandre to break through his paralysis during our first hypnotherapy session:

It is now a well-known fact that we stimulate the same brain regions when we visualize an action and when we actually perform that same action. For example, when you visualize lifting your right hand, it stimulates the same part of the brain that is activated when you actually lift your right hand . . .

When a person has a stroke due to a blood clot in a brain artery, blood cannot reach the tissue that the artery once fed with oxygen and nutrients, and that tissue dies. This tissue death then spreads to the surrounding area that does not receive the blood any more. However, if a person with this stroke imagines moving the affected arm or leg, brain blood flow to the affected area increases and the surrounding brain tissue is saved. Imagining moving a limb, even after it has been paralyzed after a stroke, increases brain blood flow enough to diminish the amount of tissue death.[4]

Witnessing a paralyzed man break through his paralysis, along with his debilitating, all-encompassing depression, changed me at the core. That day, I gave notice at my corporate job and vowed to help ease needless suffering in the world by making hypnosis mainstream. I launched my business through LivingSocial (a flash-sale company like Groupon) and sold 952 sessions in less than twenty-four hours and conducted more than a thousand private hypnotherapy sessions my first year as a hypnotherapist.

The best personal outcome from this experience? (Yes, it gets even better!) I ended up marrying Alexandre's son, Bernardo; Alex became my father-in-law.

Since then Bernardo and I have been building our company, Grace Space Hypnosis, together. Grace Space Hypnosis and Grace Space Hypnotherapy School are now the number one providers of hypnosis education, products, and services in the world. To date,

---

4 Diane Zimberoff, "Hypnosis and the Science of Visualization," *Wellness Institute Blog*, July 17, 2014, https://web.wellness-institute.org/blog/bid/391943/Hypnosis-and-the-Science-of-Visualization.

my work has been featured in the *Atlantic, Forbes, Entrepreneur, InStyle, Marie Claire*, BuzzFeed, Bustle, mindbodygreen, She-Knows, and dozens of podcasts. I am also grateful to be a recurring guest on *The Dr. Oz Show* and CBS's hit show *The Doctors*. You can visit www.gshypnosis.com/press to read all these articles and watch our TV segments.

While Bernardo and I are proud of how far we've come since that miraculous day with his dad, we didn't build all this alone. We built this company *with* our community as much as we built it *for* them. In fact, from time to time you'll notice I reference customers, clients, and hypnotherapy certification students of mine, all members of our community whom we lovingly refer to as Grace Spacers, who provided questions, testimonials, and more to support the creation of this book.

As a hypnotherapist my expertise *is* your subconscious mind—how it was programmed, how to upgrade it, why it's doing what it's doing (even if that isn't helping you), and, most important, how to condition your subconscious to *serve* you.

A Brief Introduction to Hypnosis

My first book-baby was born in 2017. Her name is *Close Your Eyes, Get Free: Use Self-Hypnosis to Reduce Stress, Quit Bad Habits, and Achieve Greater Relaxation and Focus*. She was written as the definitive guide to mastering self-hypnosis and is meant to be the foundational book from which many topic-specific books spring, of which *Close Your Eyes, Lose Weight* is the first.

I know how it can feel to read a book that feels like one big, long promotion for another book because the author keeps reiterating, "You can learn about this in my other book!" On the flip side, I also know how it can feel to read the same book twice because an author duplicates so much material from one book to the next. I will do my best to strike a balance by giving you the essentials of what you need here and by only reminding you at helpful intervals of concepts you can find in greater depth in *Close Your Eyes, Get Free*.

In the meantime, these are some of the topics covered in great detail in *Close Your Eyes, Get Free*, should you find yourself craving more in-depth information:

- how our habits are formed;
- the history of hypnosis;
- the science of hypnosis;
- my four steps to mental freedom; and
- my philosophy about how subconscious issues are formed and how to solve them by always going for the root cause.

Let's briefly review the most important aspects of what you need to know for *this* book to change your life.

If you were to put electrodes on your beautiful head to measure the brainwaves you are producing at various levels of consciousness, this is what you would find:

- beta brainwaves—normal talking, waking consciousness
- alpha brainwaves—daydreaming, lightly relaxed consciousness
- theta brainwaves—deeply relaxed, highly focused, subconsciousness
- delta brainwaves—sleep, unconsciousness

You access your subconscious mind by relaxing into what is called the "theta brainwave state." Hypnosis is how you *intentionally* enter into the theta brainwave state. Put another way, hypnosis is simply meditation with a goal. If you've ever meditated, or attempted to meditate, you know that while you may be physically and mentally relaxed during the practice, you are still aware of your surroundings and, especially early on in your practice, you are likely to have thoughts running through your mind. Hypnosis feels like meditation: a gentle, deeply relaxed state. You are still aware of your surroundings, you are in control, and you will likely continue to think some (if not many) conscious thoughts during the practice. It's important to understand that if you continue to think thoughts during hypnosis, you are still "doing it correctly," just as you would be with meditation. There is no blackout state, no amnesia, no getting stuck, no truth serum. That's all Hollywood and stage-show nonsense.

This book is written with hypnotic language sprinkled throughout so that you will read it from a state that will result in faster integration and greater memory retention of the key points. Phrases such as "take a nice, deep letting-go breath" aren't there to be cute; they intentionally help you to settle down into a lovely light hypnotic state.

According to a study published in *Psychotherapy*, researchers found that hypnotherapy outperformed both psychoanalysis and behavior therapy in terms of number of sessions required to achieve a specific result—with 93 percent recovery after six sessions for hypnotherapy, 72 percent recovery after twenty-two sessions for behavior therapy, and 38 percent recovery after six hundred sessions for psychoanalysis.[5]

Other incredible findings have shown that hypnosis therapy and treatment may do the following:

---

5 Alfred A. Barrios, "Hypnotherapy: A Reappraisal," *Psychotherapy: Theory, Research and Practice* 7, no. 1 (1970): 5.

- **Double the survival rate of breast cancer patients.**
  Women with metastatic breast cancer who received
  group hypnosis therapy were able to reduce their
  pain experience by 50 percent compared to a control group.[6] At a ten-year follow-up study of these
  same women, the hypnosis treatment group had
  double the survival rate of the control group.[7]
- **Help bones heal 40 percent faster.** Studies from
  Harvard Medical School show that hypnosis significantly reduces the time it takes to heal. Six weeks
  after an ankle fracture, those in the hypnosis group
  showed the equivalent of eight and a half weeks of
  healing.[8]
- **Demonstrate up to 80 percent success rates in
  treating irritable bowel syndrome (IBS).** Out of a
  thousand IBS patients treated with twelve sessions of hypnotherapy, 76 percent of the patients
  improved from the treatment. Success rates with
  females was 80 percent versus 62 percent with
  males.[9]
- **Lower acute and chronic pains.** A study published
  in the *Journal of General Internal Medicine* showed
  that hypnotic suggestion significantly reduced acute

6 D. Spiegel and J. R. Bloom, "Group Therapy and Hypnosis Reduce Metastatic Breast Carcinoma Pain," *Psychosomatic Medicine* 45, no. 4 (1983): 333–39.

7 D. Spiegel et al., "Effect of Psychosocial Treatment on Survival of Patients with Metastatic Breast Cancer," *Lancet* 334, no. 8668 (1989): 888–91, www.sciencedirect.com/science/article/pii/S0140673689915511.

8 "Hypnosis Helps Healing," *Harvard Gazette*, May 8, 2003, http://news.harvard.edu/gazette/2003/05.08/01-hypnosis.html.

9 V. Miller et al., "Hypnotherapy for Irritable Bowel Syndrome: An Audit of One Thousand Adult Patients," *Alimentary Pharmacology & Therapeutics* 41, no. 9 (2015): 844–55, www.ncbi.nlm.nih.gov/pubmed/25736234.

pain experienced by hospital patients.[10] A different trial showed that adding hypnosis to pain education (PE) resulted in improved outcomes over PE alone in patients with chronic nonspecific low back pain.[11]

- **Improve quality of life for children with chronic pain syndrome.** "The aim of this study was to assess the efficacy of self-hypnosis in a therapeutic education program (TEP) for the management of chronic pain in 26 children aged 7 to 17 years. Outcomes of the study were a total or a partial (at least 1) achievement of the therapeutic goals (pain, quality of sleeping, schooling, and functional activity). Sixteen patients decreased their pain intensity, 10 reached all of their therapeutic goals, and 9 reached them partially. Self-hypnosis was the only component of the TEP associated with these improvements. The current study supports the efficacy of self-hypnosis in our TEP program for chronic pain management in children."[12]

- **Help fibromyalgia patients heal from traumatic life events.** A recent study designed to determine whether hypnosis was more effective than clinical interviews in finding traumatic events in

10 University of Utah, "Mind-Body Therapies Immediately Reduce Unmanageable Pain in Hospital Patients," ScienceDaily, July 25, 2017, www.sciencedaily.com/releases/2017/07/170725122228.htm.

11 Nicholas Sterkers et al., "Hypnosis as Adjunct Therapy to Conscious Sedation for Venous Access Device Implantation in Breast Cancer: A Pilot Study," *Journal of Vascular Access* 19, no. 4 (2018), https://doi.org/10.1177/1129729818757975.

12 Honorine Delivet et al., "Efficacy of Self-Hypnosis on Quality of Life for Children with Chronic Pain Syndrome," *International Journal of Clinical and Experimental Hypnosis* 66, no. 1 (2018): 43–55, https://doi.org/10.1080/00207144.2018.1396109.

fibromyalgia patients found that "in the hypnotic state, the patients expressed 9.8 times more traumatic life events than in the waking state, a statistically significant difference with a large effect size."[13]

These studies, among countless others, show the incredible efficacy of hypnotherapy and how life changing this modality is. But despite the evidence, some still have reservations. This is understandable, given the way hypnosis has historically been represented in the media. Let's talk about how and why hypnosis is *the* most effective way for you to reprogram your subconscious.

Frequently Asked Questions

Is hypnotherapy for me?

Yes! Hypnotherapy is for just about **everyone** (see contraindications below). It is an effective, noninvasive way to improve your life. That said, as I am not a medical doctor, please know that I am not offering medical advice. I recommend you discuss your desire to use hypnosis with your primary care physician before practicing any of the exercises or before following along with any of the audio recordings provided in the online materials.

Are there any circumstances under which hypnosis is not recommended?

The only known contraindication for hypnosis or hypnotherapy at this time is schizophrenia. Even so, this book is for informational

---

13 F. X. Almeida-Marques, J. Sánchez-Blanco, and F. J. Cano-García, "Hypnosis Is More Effective than Clinical Interviews," *International Journal of Clinical and Experimental Hypnosis* 66, no. 1 (2018): 3–18, https://doi.org/10.1080/0020714 4.2018.1396104.

purposes only and is not intended to serve as a substitute for professional medical advice. As always, a health-care professional should be consulted regarding your specific medical situation.

When should I practice self-hypnosis?

For obvious reasons, never listen to hypnosis recordings while driving, operating machinery, or doing anything you wouldn't normally do while deeply relaxed. I recommend practicing self-hypnosis and listening to the provided hypnosis recordings in a safe place, which means a comfortable, quiet place where you won't be disturbed.

Is hypnosis sleep?

I realize it can be confusing when movies and stage shows employ the word *sleep* shouted out at the top of the hypnotist's lungs, followed by the client slumping over. It looks like they must be sleeping, right? Nope! Hypnosis is **not** sleep, and the client is not sleeping during a hypnotherapy session. Is it possible for a client to fall asleep during a hypnotherapy session or while listening to a recording? Yes; however, the two are mutually exclusive, and if this happens, there tends to be a simple explanation: the client was exhausted and needed a nap!

Since hypnosis is not sleep, one does not "wake up" from hypnosis. The client simply shifts from the theta brainwave state to a regular waking state of consciousness (beta brainwave).

Is a private hypnotherapy session, a hypnosis recording, or self-hypnosis more effective?

At times I will recommend, in addition to reading this book, working with a hypnotherapist simply because the topic at hand will lend itself to deeper one-on-one work. But fear not. I, too, am tired of reading books that give you the "what" but never the "how," that require you to purchase another program to experience the benefits

	Financial Investment	Speed of transformation	Average rate of efficacy per topic	Requirements for use	Time commitment per session	# of sessions/repetitions needed
Private hypnotherapy session	$$$	Fastest	★★★★	Requires a hypnotherapist and a quiet location where it is safe to close eyes for duration of the session	Approx. 45–60 minutes (specific types of sessions may be longer)	Average of 6 sessions per topic to experience at least 93% improvement per topic. Continue having sessions until you experience the result you desire.
Hypnosis recording	$	Moderately fast	★★★	Requires headphones, an audio player, and location where it is safe to close your eyes for length of recording	Varies—usually 10–60 minutes	Typically, at least 21 consecutive days of the same recording to experience at least 80% improvement per topic. Continue practicing until you experience the results you desire.
Self-hypnosis	Free	Slowest—requires the most repetition	★★★	Can be done anytime, anywhere, except while driving	Approx. 1–5 minutes	Typically, at least 90 consecutive days of the same self-hypnosis practice to experience at least 50% improvement. Continue practicing until you see the results you desire.

of the book's promise. I assure you this is not that. I guarantee you that you are going to be doing so much self-hypnosis and listening to hypnosis audios (available for free at www.CloseYourEyesLose-Weight.com) every day that lasting transformation will take place without spending a penny more.

That said, it would be a disservice if I didn't let you know when private hypnotherapy sessions would make the greatest impact on any given topic. For example, someone could be listening to a weight loss hypnosis recording with the goal of losing fifteen pounds, but then as a result of the recording discovers the subconscious is resistant to losing weight because they fear receiving more sexual attention from their spouse. There could be so much to unpack here—fear of being seen, not wanting to be intimate with their spouse, fear of intimacy altogether, deep-seated marital issues, perhaps sexual trauma, or embedded fears of being sinful from a religious upbringing. I'm sure you can see how this person will heal so much more quickly by working with a private hypnotherapist and going straight to the source of their unique challenges. So while you will receive as much support as a book and recordings can give you, I do recommend keeping in mind that working privately with a certified Grace Space hypnotherapist will help you work through, heal, and clear up any deeper issues much faster than with self-hypnosis and hypnosis audio recordings alone.

How do I work with you?

I look forward to it! Please visit www.gracesmithtv.com and follow me on Instagram @gracesmithtv to learn more about my Executive HypnoCoaching program, corporate retainer options, and speaking fees. While my personal availability is limited, I have certified and trained more than two hundred (as of the writing of this book) incredible hypnotherapists whose fees and availability are much more accessible. Read on to learn how to work with a Grace Space Hypnotherapist.

How do I work with a hypnotherapist you trained and certified?

Students who graduate at the top of their class from my Grace Space Hypnotherapy School join our team and offer phone sessions to clients anywhere in the world. Phone sessions are typically more effective than in-person sessions because you can pop on your headphones, close your eyes, and relax in your pajamas from the comfort of your own home while the sound of your hypnotherapist's voice gently upgrades your subconscious mind. Without having to rush to and from an in-person office session, the length of time you are in the theta state is extended, which means more impact for your subconscious mind. If you would like to work with a Grace Space Hypnotherapist who was personally trained by me, you can learn more and book your phone hypnotherapy sessions by visiting: www.gshypnosis.com/private-hypnotherapy-sessions.

How do I become a certified hypnotherapist?

There is no other way to say it: becoming a hypnotherapist is an incredibly rewarding career choice. Whether you would be adding the skill of hypnotherapy to an existing medical or coaching practice or are launching a brand-new career in wellness, I commend you for your interest in helping others so deeply! Grace Space Hypnotherapy School is my 250+-hour certification course that includes both online and in-person components. At the time of writing this, my students hail from all over the world, including the USA, Germany, Estonia, Costa Rica, the Cayman Islands, Singapore, the United Kingdom, Poland, and Australia. Upon successful completion of all coursework and exams, my students are certified by IACT (the International Association of Counselors and Therapists). I so look forward to your success as a certified Grace Space Hypnotherapist! For more information and to enroll, visit www.gshypnosis.com/school.

Now, let's talk about how you can use this book to reprogram your subconscious, change your habits, and experience the lasting results you're looking for!

How to Use This Book

Before you're done reading this book, you will have reprogrammed twelve core subconscious areas related to successful and lasting weight loss:

1. The fundamentals (which include chewing, proper hydration, and how to stop eating when satisfied)
2. Limiting beliefs
3. Intuitive eating
4. Exercise
5. Emotional eating
6. Eating when bored
7. Rewiring "rewards"
8. People and places to avoid
9. Visualizing what you want (using the law of attraction)
10. Unwanted attention
11. Resistance
12. Self-love

This book has been written as a ninety-day plan and includes journal sections so you can track your progress in a way that feels uplifting and supportive to you. There is a homework section at the end of each chapter that will always include at least (a) your self-hypnosis practice for the week and (b) the hypnotherapy recording for you to listen to each week. You'll notice that as this book progresses the chapters become shorter than they are in the beginning. I intentionally front-load you with information so you have everything you need to courageously dive deep into your subconscious weight loss journey knowing this will be different from any of your previous weight loss attempts. At the same time, the main promise of this book is your *results*, not providing you with a master's in physiology, psychology, or any other ology. This is much more of a *work*book than a *text*book, and because time is your most precious commodity, it's meant to give you what you need to experience the results you desire—nothing less, nothing more. Remember, the most important keys to your success will be sticking with your daily self-hypnosis practice and listening to your daily hypnosis recordings found in the free bonus section at www.CloseYourEyesLoseWeight.com.

How to Use Your Journal

It is important to track your development throughout this book for a number of reasons:

- The data will show you which areas would benefit from additional subconscious conditioning.
- The data will tell a story so you can begin to identify patterns in your behavior that you might desire to shift on the subconscious level.
- The data is valuable information you can share with your hypnotherapist (should you choose to work with one—visit www.CloseYourEyesLoseWeight.com for more info).

You will be tracking your progress each week and then graphing your summaries each month so that you will have a visual representation of your progress in each of the twelve key areas we will work on in this book. Consider the following ways in which you can track your weight loss success and choose the method that works best for you.

Tracking Physical Weight Loss

If you feel you'll get the most out of this program by getting on a scale each morning and tracking your weight, this section is for you. According to the Centers for Disease Control and Prevention (CDC), it is safe to lose one to two pounds per week. That means, on average, aiming for four to eight pounds of weight loss per month is a healthy goal.[14] Using the CDC's guidelines, by the end of the ninety days you can safely lose between sixteen and thirty-two pounds. In other words, it's not helpful to declare a goal of losing forty-five pounds in the first month, since that is thirteen pounds more than the high-end figure recommended by the CDC.

If your goal is to lose more than thirty-two pounds in total, after the first ninety days are complete you can continue your journey by repeating this program and taking each one of these lessons deeper (as you'll see in chapter two, the most powerful hypno-affirmations are **achievable** and **believable**, so set realistic goals, set yourself up for success, and keep moving toward your ultimate goal as you reach milestones). Using the CDC's guidelines, after two rounds you can safely lose up to sixty-four pounds—and that's only six months into a brand-new life. In one year, that's up to 128 pounds lost!

Remember, this is not a fad diet or a race to the finish line. You're rewiring your brain. That takes time. Happily, hypnosis rewires the brain much faster than any other means (see page 25 in chapter two for more on this), while still conditioning you for a

---

14 Rena Goldman, "How Much Weight Can You Lose in a Month?," Healthline, July 27, 2016, www.healthline.com/health/food-nutrition/weight-loss-in-a-month.

new lifestyle for the rest of your life. We care about lasting results and forming the beliefs that will support your empowered, healthy choices in the long run. So when setting your weekly, monthly, and ninety-day goals, please keep those numbers in mind. For those with a history of disordered eating, tracking your weight every day might lead to obsessive-compulsive behavior or negativity. If that is the case, please know yourself, remember to consult with your doctor, and choose to track your progress through less triggering means—for example, through energy levels and how you feel in your clothes.

If you choose to use your daily weight as a metric for progress, please keep in mind that your weight will be affected by the amount of water you will soon be drinking. Also keep in mind that muscle weighs more than fat! So if you see the number on the scale going up a bit one week, but your measurement for how you feel in your clothes is improving, you can ascertain from the data that you are losing fat and gaining muscle mass, so you're still headed in the direction you want. Be your own best advocate when choosing how to track your progress. Turn to page 52 to get a glimpse of how you'll track your weight each day.

Tracking Measurements

If you prefer to track your measurements (inches lost, rather than pounds lost) keep in mind that "on average, for every 8.5 pounds lost, people dropped an inch off their waist."[15] So if you would like to lose thirty pounds over the course of ninety days, that will be approximately 3.5 inches off your waistline, and so on. You can see the simple chart below for reference.

---

15 "What Size Will You Be After You Lose Weight?," Decision Science News, November 14, 2014, www.decisionsciencenews.com/2014/11/14/size-will-lose -weight/.

Pounds Lost	10	20	30	40	50	60	70	80	90	100	110	120	130	140	150
Approx. Inches Dropped Off Waist	1.2	2.4	3.5	4.7	5.9	7.1	8.2	9.1	10.6	11.8	12.9	14.1	15.3	16.5	17.6

In the journal pages, there is space for you to track the measurements of your neck, chest, arms, hip, waist, and thighs. Track the measurements of all of these areas, some of them, or none of them. Again, only use this method of tracking if it feels empowering to you. Turn to page 52 to take a look at how you'll track each day.

Other Ways to Track Your Success

You can also track your daily **energy levels** and how you feel in your **clothes**. These are less triggering ways to notice your improvements, but they are also less concrete. Energy levels are either low, medium, or high. They are not your emotions (happy, sad, etc.) but rather how energetic you feel, regardless of your emotions. Do your clothes feel tight, comfortable, or loose? These options are typically comfortable for most and are a nice way to reassociate weight loss progress with positive emotions and feelings. Turn to page 52 to see what tracking these daily will look like.

What Is Healthy Versus What Is Helpful

This book is not here to make moral judgments. Everyone, at any size, is worthy and deserving of love and respect! In *Body Positive Power*, body-empowerment author Megan Jayne Crabbe writes,

> The relationship between health and weight is not what we think it is, and the assumptions we currently hold are hurting us all, fat, thin, and every size in between. And most importantly, whatever we might believe about size,

fitness, weight, and health doesn't really matter when it comes to body positivity. Because physical health is not a requirement for self-love, respect, or to be treated with basic human dignity. Those are things that we all deserve, regardless of how our bodies look or how our bodies function.[16]

This book is for those empowered folks who've decided they'd like to lose weight, for the right reasons. Learning to fall in love with yourself, as you are *today*, is a key component in why you will experience success with this program when you haven't before. It's not just about learning to eat "healthy." Yes, from time to time I might write a phrase like "eat healthy," but the truth is, what is "healthy" can often be deceiving. I reached out to Maggie Berghoff, a world-renowned nurse practitioner specializing in functional medicine, to get her perspective on this trend I've noticed again and again with my clients: what's "healthy" for one is sometimes terrible for another.

Maggie said: "We have access to some of the most cutting-edge technology and knowledge now to identify exactly what is most 'healthy' for your specific body. We can look at your pathways, genetics, biomarkers, and current internal health status to determine what will best get you the health and wellness results you're looking for, in the most foolproof way . . . Gone are the days when 'one size fits all' diet plans are the only option."[17] Maggie used lemon water as an example. Drinking lemon water is often touted as a "healthy habit" to lose weight and detoxify, and while it may be helpful and

16 Megan Jayne Crabbe, *Body Positive Power* (New York: Seal Press, 2018), 197–98.

17 Maggie Berghoff, email message to the author, October 26, 2019. See maggieberghoff.com for more advice from Maggie.

anti-inflammatory to some people, it can cause more harm than good to others (e.g., those with heartburn or citrus allergies).

In my own personal experience of healing "leaky gut" (more about this on page 115), I went from being able to eat anything to having severe allergic reactions to celery, almonds, ginger, broccoli, and other extremely healthy foods. Being doubled over with pain and nausea doesn't feel healthy! There were days when all I could eat was "junk food." My body wouldn't attack pizza. Go figure. Still, that pizza wasn't "healthy" even though it didn't make me instantly sick, and I gained weight as a result.

Since what's "healthy" is more subjective than we might have once thought, more often than not, I'll be referring to choices that are either *helpful* to you as they relate to your weight loss goals, or unhelpful to you, rather than what is healthy or unhealthy. Sitting on the couch and eating chips is unhelpful to anyone's weight loss goals, full stop. My aim in this book is to be inclusive and empowering without treading so lightly on eggshells for fear of upsetting or triggering one particular kind of reader that the efficacy of the book is diminished for all other readers. It's not the simplest line to toe because this can be such an inflammatory subject, but it's a worthwhile and important one, so I hope what you find beyond this point will lift you up, make you think, and challenge old, unhelpful patterns. After all, the title of this book is *Close Your Eyes, Lose Weight*—so let's get started helping you effectively, naturally, and noninvasively lose the weight you want to lose!

PART I

Preparing for Your 90-Day Program

CHAPTER 1

. . . .

Why Was It So Darn Hard to Lose Weight in the Past?

After her children went to sleep, Susan sat on the couch and scrolled through countless TV channels. It took her so long to choose what to watch that her husband, Jim, gave up and went to bed in a huff. Susan wondered if she was indecisive because she knew it annoyed Jim. Because she wanted to have some control in "his" house.

But deep down, Susan knew the scrolling numbed her. That's what she wanted. If she was too alert, too aware, the thoughts would come: Is this all there is? Will I always feel like this? Always look like this? Am I passing this on to my kids?

Susan felt riddled with guilt. Why wasn't she grateful? Her three kids, twelve-year-old Sammy, eight-year-old Josephine, and six-year-old Michael, were healthy and happy. Jim had a steady foreman job that more than covered their bills. Susan got to be a stay-at-home mom and volunteer on the weekends. What more could she ask for?

Yet she had felt defeated physically, emotionally, mentally, and even spiritually for a long time. She felt like her body was a silent enemy she'd carry around forever. The extra seventy-two pounds, aching joints, rolls, sciatica, diabetes, and high blood pressure tormented her. She didn't want to think about them. So she scrolled and scrolled . . .

One night, in the middle of her channel-surfing routine, Susan saw a book on the coffee table out of the corner of her eye.

"Susie, just read it!" her sister-in-law had exclaimed as she thrust the book at her earlier that day. "I'm down eight pounds, and it hasn't been a month. Don't roll your eyes at me. You'll love it." And she had tossed the book onto the coffee table on her way out the door.

Susan sighed. Nothing to watch. What do I have to lose? She picked up *Close Your Eyes, Lose Weight*, pulled her blanket closer, and began to read . . .

. . . .

You are no doubt holding this book in your hands because you have been struggling to lose weight. Because nothing else has worked with the lasting results you desire. And you're not alone. Over the years, I have worked with thousands of clients with all sorts of goals—to run a 5k, to feel more confident in the boardroom, to land an audition, or to stop being so triggered by other people's opinions . . . Of the myriad areas they would like to work on, nearly 90 percent of my clients say, "Oh, and if I could lose an extra ten pounds, that would be great." In other words, no matter what my clients came to me for, nine out of ten also wanted to lose weight as a "cherry on top."

Of course, there are also clients who come to hypnosis specifically to lose a significant amount of weight, even a hundred pounds or more.

What this indicates is that almost no one is happy with their weight.

Almost no one is happy with their size.

Almost no one is happy with their body.

While the body positivity movement is thankfully gaining strength, there are still millions of people, mostly women, diagnosed with anorexia, bulimia, or disordered eating each year.

According to the National Association of Anorexia Nervosa and Associated Disorders (ANAD):

- At least thirty million people of all ages and genders suffer from an eating disorder in the United States.
- Every sixty-two minutes at least one person dies as a direct result of an eating disorder.
- Eating disorders have the highest mortality rate of any mental illness.[18]

And the American Academy of Child & Adolescent Psychiatry states, "In the United States, as many as 10 in 100 young women suffer from an eating disorder."[19]

---

18 "Eating Disorder Statistics," ANAD, https://anad.org/education-and -awareness/about-eating-disorders/eating-disorders-statistics/.

19 "Eating Disorders in Teens," American Academy of Child & Adolescent Psychiatry, March 2018, www.aacap.org/AACAP/Families_and_Youth/Facts_for_ Families/FFF-Guide/Teenagers-With-Eating-Disorders-002.aspx.

The Importance of Body Positivity

Even though I have helped thousands of clients and customers lose weight with hypnosis, I was nervous about writing this book. I was nervous it might appear that I believe—or that this book might contribute to the cultural discourse and belief—that one has to look a certain way to earn love and acceptance. I do not believe that, not for one second. I believe that being healthy, happy, and free is the goal. This can be achieved in so many shapes and sizes. Feeling unhealthy, depressed, and caged in is causing human beings to live less fulfilling lives than the ones they deserve to live. The only thing *I* want is for you to learn how to access your subconscious mind so you can do and think and feel what *you* want to do and think and feel. To reject what others want for you and what their conditioning is keeping you from experiencing—your freedom.

I hope you want to fall in love with your magnificence, which is not something you can buy, because you are *already* magnificent. Hypnosis can help you to accept and own that truth. I hope you want to stop hiding for fear of judgment, for fear of attention, for fear of being too much, for fear of being not enough. Hypnosis can help you do that by building up your self-worth, self-love, and self-confidence, which are your birthrights. I hope you want to stop feeling like you have to apologize for being who you are. Hypnosis can help you do that by reinforcing that your uniqueness (including your physical body) is your superpower. I hope you want to experience what *mental freedom* is and know that you are worthy and deserving of having it. Hypnosis can help you experience these things because each and every one of them live in your subconscious mind, and hypnosis is the most natural, noninvasive, and effective way to access your subconscious.

My interest is not in weight loss per se. My interest is you being in control of your life, your thoughts, your emotions, *your* body.

I share this because first and foremost I want to lift humanity *up*, not participate in rhetoric that drags us down, and a culture obsessed with impossible beauty standards drags us down.

I've noticed that over the past two years, although I have as many clients who want to lose weight as before, quite a few of my clients now express **shame** for wanting to lose weight at all. In desiring to honor all things wonderful and woke, something developed for many of my clients: they came in experiencing shame for having a body that was bigger than they thought it should be, but they now also had the added shame for wanting to lose weight at all. To even desire to lose weight now felt like a betrayal toward all the wonderful body positivity progress that had so painstakingly begun to make headway.

I've had clients tell me they feel trapped inside a body that isn't theirs, that the extra weight they carry is an emotional burden as much as it is a physical one, and that they want nothing more than to be free from this "prison" they live inside. Weight loss for them *is* an act of empowerment, of self-love! I've also had clients who say they want to lose fifteen pounds because their boyfriend keeps telling them they look fat when they are objectively thin. There is no way weight loss would be empowering for this person; it would add physical injury to what are emotionally abusive relationship and low self-esteem issues. The self-love, hydration, reward, and other aspects of this book would still be healing for that client, but for her, deciding she *doesn't* need to lose weight at all is where she will find her power. Everyone's reasons for being here are different. The ways you'll integrate the information found on the following pages will be different, too. Perhaps you desire to lose over a hundred pounds because three generations of women in your family have been morbidly obese and you want to break that chain. To shed all the physical and emotional challenges that have come along with all that extra weight for generations and to free future generations from the same challenges. If that's your motivation, that is beautiful, and you are worthy and deserving of not only pursuing it but of succeeding at it! Your success will lift you up, both internally and externally, emotionally and physically, consciously and subconsciously, mentally and spiritually.

Or perhaps as you work your way through this book and learn to fall in love with your body, your initial goals will change. For example, at the start the conscious mind (which has been conditioned by weight loss culture) could be saying it needs to lose fifty pounds to be worthy of love and respect. (Which is bs. You are worthy of love and respect, right now, at any size, every minute of every day, forever.) As you read this book, that old goal might shift as you come to these realizations:

1. I notice I feel sluggish, and I want more energy.
2. I know deep down in my soul that at least thirty pounds on my body are emotional, and I don't want or need to carry around that emotional baggage anymore.
3. I've been eating foods I don't want to eat because I didn't know how to process my emotions. I want that to stop.

It would be disempowering *not* to transform all of the above, even though, yes, you are worthy of love and respect just as you are right now. By reading this book, you'll make sure that, however much weight you desire to lose, the reasons for *why* you'll desire to lose them will finally be coming from a subconscious place of empowerment rather than a place of shame or societal pressure.

So let's draw the line in the sand here because no shame, old or new, is allowed from this point forward (and I'll help you release it). You're holding this book because you've decided you want to lose weight, and since your opinion is the only one that matters, your decision is an awesome one. Because you want to lose weight, we are going to pull out the stops and do whatever it takes to help you get the relationship with food, exercise, and self-love you deserve to have. Now, let's work together to make sure you're doing it for the right subconscious reasons (for *you*, from an empowered place), in a way that will have a lasting impact and that will leave you feeling happier and more in love with your own magnificence.

Weight Loss Problems Your Subconscious Mind Can Fix

Problem #1: Certain foods are naturally or have been engineered to be addictive

Certain foods release neurochemicals in your brain that make you feel oh-so-happy—oh-so-momentarily. This is why emotional eating, or eating your feelings, is the most prevalent challenge expressed by my weight loss clients. When you feel sad, you unconsciously seek out foods that will briefly release the same "feel-good" neurochemicals as addictive drugs.

According to a study by researchers at the University of Michigan, these are the top eighteen foods that participants reported as prompting the most addiction-like eating behaviors:[20]

1. Chocolate
2. Ice cream
3. French fries
4. Pizza
5. Cookies
6. Chips
7. Cake
8. Popcorn (buttered)

---

20 Erica M. Schulte, N. M. Avena, and A. N. Gearhardt, "Which Foods May Be Addictive? The Roles of Processing, Fat Content, and Glycemic Load," *PLoS One* 10, no. 2 (2015), www.ncbi.nlm.nih.gov/pubmed/25692302.

9. Cheeseburger   14. Soda (not diet)
10. Muffin   15. Rolls (plain)
11. Breakfast cereal   16. Cheese
12. Gummy candy   17. Pretzels
13. Fried chicken   18. Bacon

Do any of these look familiar, particularly when you're feeling emotional? The solution to overcoming this problem resides in your ability to reprogram your subconscious mind to process your emotions in ways that are healthy and which promote genuine long-term contentment, rather than an artificial and fleeting dopamine spike that triggers a never-ending cycle of wanting more. To break this cycle of craving foods that have been engineered to be addictive, the subconscious mind has to decide that these foods are not rewards and to not seek them when celebrating, looking for refuge, or to feel better. We will cover this in depth in chapter ten.

Problem #2: Stress makes it extremely difficult to release weight

Researchers from Yale University discovered that the "stress hormone" cortisol triggers excessive abdominal fat deposits. Stress has long been known to trigger the desire to eat more, which exacerbates weight gain by increasing caloric intake, but these findings showed, for the first time, that the secretion of cortisol was associated with both chronic stress and an increase of abdominal "belly fat."

Chronic stress also slows fat metabolism and makes it difficult to lose weight because of the production of betatrophin, which inhibits an enzyme required for fat metabolism.[21] So stress

21 Christopher Bergland, "Why Does Chronic Stress Make Losing Weight More Difficult?," *Psychology Today*, January 8, 2016, www.psychologytoday.com/intl /blog/the-athletes-way/201601/why-does-chronic-stress-make-losing-weight -more-difficult?amp.

triggers us to eat more, increases belly fat, *and* blocks the body's ability to burn fat.

If that wasn't daunting enough, unfortunately, stress is on the rise.

> According to the American Psychological Association (APA), "most Americans are suffering from moderate to high stress, with 44 percent reporting that their stress levels have increased over the past five years. Concerns about money, work and the economy top the list of most frequently cited sources of stress."[22] In a 2018 study, the APA found that stress levels among those from Generation Z (i.e., currently aged fifteen to twenty-one, who are typically in high school or college) are notably high: "Results indicate that almost a third are stressed about basic elements and necessities of life such as money and debt, housing stability, and hunger, too. Over 90 percent of respondents had stress symptoms with over half being depressed and lacking both energy and motivation."[23]

The good news is, hypnosis drastically decreases stress and anxiety levels, no matter what you're working on during your hypnotherapy session. While you'll be focused on losing weight,

22 R. A. Clay, "Stressed in America," *American Psychological Association* 42, no. 1 (2011), www.apa.org/monitor/2011/01/stressed-america.
23 Thomas G. Plante, "Americans Are Stressed Out, and It Is Getting Worse," *Psychology Today*, December 3, 2018, www.psychologytoday.com/us/blog/do-the-right-thing/201812/americans-are-stressed-out-and-it-is-getting-worse.

simply by being in the theta brainwave state (return to page xxi of the preface for a refresher on the theta brainwave state), your stress levels will decrease dramatically. Long-term use of hypnosis rewires the brain to not get as stressed in the first place, thus ending stress-related eating, belly fat, and impaired fat metabolism (more on this in chapter eight).

Problem #3: When people subconsciously hate themselves, they take actions all day long to punish themselves, because that's what they subconsciously feel they deserve

People who love themselves naturally and intuitively have a desire to take care of themselves through helpful choices. That doesn't sound like a problem, right? Except, how many people do you know who act like they love themselves? Not an egoic, overcompensating, outward display of confidence but a genuine, down-to-earth feeling of love and compassion toward oneself? Having worked with thousands of individual clients, I can tell you that it would be rare for someone to arrive to their first session with genuine self-love. After a lifetime of being hard on yourself, cultivating kind, helpful, and loving habits in the subconscious mind will have a dramatic impact on more than your health improvement goals; this will drastically improve your entire life.

How, When, and Why Did the Problems Begin?

Your subconscious mind has been imprinted with information on how to survive in this world since you were a child. The problem with this, of course, is that the information you were provided with as a child was incomplete. It was mostly given to you by people who also were never taught to upgrade the subconscious programming that was given to them by their parents, and their parents' parents, and so on, for generations back. It is important to understand that the subconscious always believes it's helping you, whether or not it is.

The following examples represent experiences and themes that I've seen again and again with my hypnotherapy clients over the years.

- At thirty-five-years old Karyn was worried she wasn't skinny enough and she would audibly express this in front of her then-five-year-old daughter, Alice. Now, Alice is thirty-five years old, and in recent months has developed an obsession over the idea that she is not skinny enough. She has no idea that she's expressing a subconscious belief she learned as a child that "thirty-five-year-old moms in our family aren't skinny enough and should stress about it out loud." Alice's subconscious is simply parroting what she learned from her mother and "provided" that extra weight right on cue at age thirty-four and a half so Alice would have it there to complain about by age thirty-five.
- Tim's dad drank beer every weekend for his entire life. Now Tim wants to stop drinking empty calories, and he's tired of feeling hungover on Monday mornings, but he feels guilty not drinking beer with his dad. He wants to continue bonding with his father on the weekends and doesn't want his dad to feel like he's judging his behavior.
- Jocelyn's grandmother was the only unconditionally loving person toward her in her family, and they would bake cookies together at the holidays. Now,

whenever Jocelyn feels sad, she "inexplicably" takes a trip to the bakery a few blocks away.

- Everyone in Doug's family ate fast while growing up. No one ever chewed their food thoroughly. Even though his new girlfriend points out how fast he eats at every meal, he feels like it's out of his control.

- Everyone in the Johnson family is overweight and, perhaps as a response to the bullying they themselves received as children, now often put down and make jokes about skinny people. For a member of the Johnson family, it would be a subconscious betrayal to become one of "them." How do you think that makes the youngest Johnson feel? He wants to grow up and be a dietitian. He's motivated to help his family, but his subconscious is terrified of being kicked out of the "tribe" for being different.

Do any of these resonate with you? If beliefs or experiences like these live in your subconscious mind, know that it is not your fault. They were put there by someone else whose subconscious mind also picked them up from someone else, likely when they were under the age of seven. In hypnotherapy we don't waste precious time pointing fingers. It's not your fault that limiting beliefs exist, but it is your responsibility to learn how to access your subconscious mind so you can change and upgrade these limiting beliefs, since you—and you alone—are the only one who can do anything about them. In other words, no one else can upgrade your subconscious mind for you.

That being said, I'm here to help as your guide, and I'll stand beside you and hold your hand as *you* make these powerful and lasting changes for yourself. Now it's time to get to the good stuff . . . the solutions.

The Solutions

These are the subconscious solutions you will master through this book:

1. You will stop living at the mercy of the neurochemicals released in the brain by foods that have been engineered to be addictive. When you use what you learn here to recondition your subconscious mind, emotional eating will cease.
2. You will release emotional weight because you will learn to turn off the flight, fight, freeze survival mechanisms (i.e., stop living in a perpetual state of stress and fear) and because you will learn to let go of shame.
3. You will learn to intuitively make the right food and lifestyle choices because you will learn to fall in love with yourself. When you love and respect yourself, subconscious self-sabotage and punishment through unhelpful choices stop.

Homework

Before moving on to chapter two, your homework is to master a technique I will refer to throughout this book. It is my favorite way to catch old negative thoughts and defuse their power.

It's simple: If you catch yourself thinking an unhelpful thought, immediately say or think, "Cancel, cancel!" Follow it with a thought that moves you in the direction of your desired life.

For example, Julie has the thought, "Ugh, I'm so fat! I look so ugly in this. I don't even want to go to this stupid event." To defuse the power of these words and to stop them from strengthening the neural pathway of this belief in the brain, Julie will say, "Cancel, cancel! I am so grateful for my beating heart, for my eyes that can see, for my ears that can hear music. My body truly is miraculous. I'm excited to dress it up tonight with an outfit that feels great."

Now, it's your turn:

1. Imagine an unhelpful thought.
2. Quickly say or think, "Cancel, cancel!"
3. Think a thought that represents how you *want* to feel or what you *want* to think instead. Make it *believable*. For example, switching from "I look fat" to "I look gorgeous" might not feel at all believable in the moment, but switching from "I look fat" to "I am so grateful for my beating heart, my body is truly miraculous" would likely feel true and empowering.

This "Cancel, cancel!" tool will help you clean your mindset of all negative thoughts and fill it up with thoughts that are in alignment with the life you desire to create. To upgrade the impact of this pattern interrupt, add a hair tie around your wrist and anytime you think an unhelpful thought, snap the band (not too hard! you're interrupting a pattern, not punishing yourself), say or think, "Cancel, cancel!" and then immediately think a helpful thought that supports you. I am constantly using "Cancel, cancel!" A negative thought rarely lingers long enough for it to stick in my mind. This homework assignment will do the same for you.

Susan's Story, Continued . . .

Three months had gone by since Susan first read *Close Your Eyes, Lose Weight*. That first night, which had started off in such a bleak yet predictable manner, had ended with Susan feeling something she hadn't felt in decades: hope. Now when Susan asks herself, "Is it possible to have more?" the answer is an emphatic yes!

"Is it possible for me to feel good?" Yes!

"Is it possible for me to feel confident?" Yes!

"Am I worthy of having more than this?" Yes!

And because her answers had changed, her actions had, too. She realized she had never taken pride in much of anything her entire life, always wanting to be humble and not braggadocious. But upon some digging into her subconscious, Susan had learned she did in fact have one area that generated all her self-respect: cooking. It was the only time Jim or the kids showed her any appreciation at all. She had been self-sabotaging her ability to make even the slightest headway into a healthier lifestyle because her sense of self-worth was tied to heaping plates of carbs and cheese and meat, deep fried or lathered in butter or sugar. The issues she had with her body and weight ran so deep that the answer wasn't simply exercising and eating less. She had to disconnect her sense of self-worth from cooking these meals that had been passed down to her from her mother and her mother's mother. In these three months, she's lost twenty-four pounds and has stopped scrolling through the TV at night. But more important, Susan now feels courageous and inspired. At night she now reads travel guides because she's got a new long-term goal—to taste-test "helpful" cuisine all over the world and bring those recipes back for her friends and family to enjoy.

CHAPTER 2

· · · · · · · · · · · · · · · · ·

How to Hypnotize Yourself for Weight Loss

"I was severely depressed, unemployed, and living in my parents' basement. My mental and physical health had deteriorated so much that I could hardly get out of bed. I found Grace's twenty-one-day hypnosis sessions and started doing it each morning and evening. I stayed consistent each day and focused on self-healing. Within months of believing it was possible to change, I started my dream job, had a new car, and moved into an incredible house with breathtaking views." –Melody S., Dolores, Colorado

This book is more than a book. It is a program complete with journal pages, audio recordings, and homework assignments. The text itself is here for you to understand why each of these twelve pillars is a necessary step to rewiring your relationship with food, your body, and your self-worth. However, the real transformation comes not from just reading the text, but from *doing the hypnosis*. Throughout this ninety-day journey, you are going to practice hypnosis four times a day. Count 'em . . . One, two, three, four! Every day, four times per day. Three times will be with the **self**-hypnosis practice I'll teach you in this chapter, so it's important to get it right! And the remaining practice will be listening to the hypnosis audio recording for each corresponding chapter. You can find them all at www. CloseYourEyesLoseWeight.com.

> The self-hypnosis process taught in this book is also slightly more streamlined than the techniques I taught in *Close Your Eyes, Get Free*, so even if you read my first book, you're going to love learning this even more efficient format.

It's the moment you've been waiting for! It's time for you to learn how to hypnotize yourself. I recommend reading through the following steps two to three times before following along so you'll have a good idea of the steps before you close your eyes. If you need to peek your eyes open to double-check the next step, that's no problem at all. I also have a video tutorial waiting for you at www. CloseYourEyesLoseWeight.com, so if you would like to watch that first, you can head there now.

How to Hypnotize Yourself

1. Notice your current stress level (0 = total relaxation, 10 = panic attack).
2. Hold your book up at a diagonal (so that it's hovering right over where the wall and ceiling meet) and read your hypno-affirmation, which is, "I am safe, I am calm. I choose to be here," over and over until you've memorized it.
3. Put your book down, place your hands comfortably in your lap, and close your eyes.
4. Say a color you love out loud (or silently in your mind) and imagine the color flowing in through the top of your head, all the way down through your body, out through the bottoms of your feet, and down into the center of the earth.
5. *Try* to open your eyelids, and notice they don't want to open.
6. Say a color you love out loud (or silently in your mind) and imagine the color flowing in through the top of your head, all the way down through your body, out the bottoms of your feet, and down into the center of the earth.
7. Count backward slowly, saying,
    "Ten, I am going deeper and deeper."
    "Nine, I am going deeper and deeper."
    "Eight, I am going deeper and deeper."
    "Seven, I am going deeper and deeper."
    "Six, I am going deeper and deeper."
    "Five, I am going deeper and deeper."
    "Four, I am going deeper and deeper."
    "Three, I am going deeper and deeper."

"Two, I am going deeper and deeper."

"One, I am going deeper and deeper."

8. Say a color you love out loud (or silently in your mind) and imagine the color flowing in through the top of your head, all the way down through your body, out the bottoms of your feet, and down into the center of the earth.

9. Repeat your hypno-affirmation (the one you memorized earlier while holding the book up at a diagonal) twenty-one times.

10. Say a color you love out loud (or silently in your mind) and imagine the color flowing in through the top of your head, all the way down through your body, out the bottoms of your feet, and down into the center of the earth.

11. Visualize the outcome you desire using all your senses (see it, hear it, touch it, taste it, smell it).

12. Say a color you love out loud (or silently in your mind) and imagine the color flowing in through the top of your head, all the way down through your body, out through the bottoms of your feet, and down into the center of the earth.

13. Open your eyes.

14. Smile to release a hit of endorphins, serotonin, and dopamine (which train your brain that you enjoyed this and want to do it again soon!).

15. Notice your new lower level (remember, 0 = total relaxation).

Great job! It's likely that you're feeling much more relaxed now. In fact, the likelihood is that you're at least 50 percent more relaxed already (see page 30 for more on this). I am so proud of you and so excited for you! Of course, it can be challenging to learn a process that requires you to close your eyes, while reading. :) For that reason, be sure to visit www.CloseYourEyesLoseWeight.com to follow along with the free video tutorial that will walk you through this process. In no time at all, you'll be a self-hypnosis pro.

Here is a summary of what you learned:

1. Notice starting number
2. Hold book up
3. Close your eyes
4. Run the color
5. Try the eyes
6. Run the color
7. Count down
8. Run the color
9. Hypno-affirmation × 21
10. Run the color
11. Visualize
12. Run the color
13. Open eyes
14. Smile
15. Notice new number

You'll notice that once you close your eyes, "Run the color" happens before and after every single new step, so this process is actually *very easy* to memorize. The only steps you have to remember while your eyes are closed are "try the eyes," "count down," "hypno-affirmation x 21," and "visualize." If you're in a pinch for time, you can shorten this process in the following way:

1. Notice starting number
2. Hold book up
3. Close your eyes
4. Run the color
5. Try the eyes
6. Run the color
7. ~~Count down~~
8. ~~Run the color~~
9. Hypno-affirmation *~~21~~* 3
10. ~~Run the color~~
11. ~~Visualize~~
12. Run the color
13. Open eyes
14. Smile
15. Notice new number

To summarize, you remove the countdown (step seven), run the color (step eight), repeat your hypno-affirmation three times instead of twenty-one times (step nine), run the color (step ten), and also remove the visualization step (step eleven). This shorter version is only to be done when your time is limited. The standard practice is much more effective as far as conditioning goes, which you want since it will upgrade your self-hypnosis tool from being prescriptive to being preventive much faster than the shorter version. Still, some hypnosis is always better than no hypnosis! I'd much rather you use the shortened version than none at all. Just use the standard practice more often than not.

More Frequently Asked Questions

Take a nice, deep letting-go breath. Now that you've learned how to do self-hypnosis, allow me to answer all the frequently asked questions we receive about this life-changing technique.

Why is it important to practice self-hypnosis three times per day?

Great question. The short answer is: the more you practice self-hypnosis, the faster it goes from being *prescriptive* to being *preventive.*

When someone is sick, a doctor often prescribes medicine to make them feel better, to alleviate the symptoms. The prescription usually isn't solving the root of the issue and usually isn't preventing the issue from returning again in the future. It is a welcomed bandage that provides short-term support and comfort. In the beginning, self-hypnosis is *prescriptive.* You have it handy to help you when you're feeling angry, stressed out, or afraid and can use it to change your state in a few minutes. It's common to be able to go from an eight to a two on the stress scale (more on this in a bit) with one or two rounds of self-hypnosis. This in and of itself is life transforming.

However, what's even more incredible is that, with enough practice, self-hypnosis goes from being prescriptive to being *preventive.* Preventive medicine wards off the possibility of the issue developing in the first place so we won't need a bandage of relief later on. With enough self-hypnosis, you're conditioning your brain to stay much calmer with increasing regularity. With time that could mean that your new peak stress level is perhaps a six or a four instead of an eight, which is more manageable and supportive of all areas of your life.

What are hypno-affirmations?

Hypno-affirmation is a word I use to describe what hypnotherapists usually refer to as "suggestions." I found that most of my clients were familiar with the idea of repeating positive, daily affirmations and that the term "hypno-affirmation" made the parallel between these two practices clear. With hypno-affirmations we are using positive phrases (that are easy to remember) to condition the subconscious mind. Hypno-affirmations are infinitely more powerful than affirmations alone as they reach the subconscious mind directly, without the massive impediment of the conscious mind standing in the way. The self-hypnosis **process** will stay the same throughout this book; the only parts that **change** are the **hypno-affirmations** with each chapter.

You might be wondering how hypno-affirmations differ from traditional affirmations. Daily affirmations can be fabulous, but they only reach the *conscious* mind. It takes a long, *long* time for them to influence your subconscious. Anyone who has practiced them knows it. You might feel better for a short time, but the underlying issue remains unless you repeat those bad boys an average of six hundred times per day for a week (at least). Typically, people give up well before that happens.

The difference here is that we use hypno-affirmations during self-hypnosis, which means you are in the theta brainwave state during the conditioning process. Because you are repeating the hypno-affirmations to your *sub*conscious mind, much less repetition is required. Usually ten to twenty-one repetitions per day does the trick. This is the difference between taking a rowboat to get where you're going and taking a private jet. Affirmations on their own might get you there, but hypno-affirmations used during self-hypnosis sessions are a much faster and more direct ride.

The hypno-affirmation you used during your first practice round was "I am safe, I am calm. I choose to be here." It's a beautiful catchall hypno-affirmation because it works in every situation to make you feel better.

- **"I am safe."** Affirming this turns survival mode *off*. The fight, flight, freeze sensations that come from the feeling of "danger" dissipate. Remember from chapter one (page 10) that these feelings produce cortisol, the hunger-inducing, belly fat–producing, metabolic-blocking hormone? If you feel safe, you produce less cortisol. Also, as you'll see later, feeling safe naturally cuts down on emotional eating and binging tendencies.

- **"I am calm."** This affirms what you *want*. Most people go around talking about how stressed they are and how much anxiety they have all day long. Does talking about feeling stress get rid of it? Or does it strengthen those neurological pathways and create more stress and anxiety? You guessed it! Talking about how stressed you are makes you more stressed. When was the last time you affirmed how you *wanted* to feel instead? This hypno-affirmation will train your brain to focus on what you do want, not what you don't want.

- **"I choose to be here."** This is a bit of a mystical double entendre. *I choose to be here* can mean that you choose to be sitting in *this* meeting, driving in *this* traffic, having *this* dentist appointment. It takes away the subconscious panic from perceived lack of control. *I **choose** to be here* brings calm and confidence because it affirms you have a choice—you are in control—and this is what *you* chose. It can also mean *I choose to be **here***—that is, in the present moment. All worrying takes place when your mind wanders into either the past or the future. Peace is found right here in the only time that exists: the present moment. Find it by choosing to be *here*.

How to Write Your Own Hypno-affirmations

In addition to "I am safe, I am calm. I choose to be here," I'll also be providing you with a myriad of hypno-affirmations written specifically for the twelve subconscious areas of weight loss at the end of each chapter. In addition to these, if you would ever like to write your own hypno-affirmations in the future, use the following guidelines:

- **Desirable.** This is the most important factor. If you don't want the result, you're not going to get it. Hypnosis is not mind control. It cannot make you do what you don't want to do. Imagine a scale of desirability: zero means you don't want it at all; ten means you want it more than anything in the world. Hypnosis becomes effective when you are at a level of seven or above. So if you're losing weight because someone *else* wants you to (a level five at highest), I'd lovingly suggest you gift this book to a friend who is at a level seven or above on the desirability scale and focus your energies on using hypnosis to get a result you desire for something else you want!

- **Achievable and Believable.** If you want $1 million but you earned $100,000 last year, your subconscious will sniff out an "I am a millionaire" hypno-affirmation, stamp it as "bs," and return to its abundance-self-sabotage-business-as-usual. You can have any desired outcome you want if you work up to it so the subconscious doesn't mark it as "impossible" before you even get started. If you'd like to lose a hundred pounds, you already know that's not achievable, believable, or even safe within our ninety-day format. Can you do it eventually? Heck yes. You can also earn a million dollars! But make sure your first hypno-affirmations are achievable and believable and then ramp them up as you meet your milestones. If losing a hundred pounds is your ultimate goal, make your hypno-affirmations supportive of losing twenty-four pounds in your first round of this ninety-day program. In one short year from today, you'll have achieved your goal, and you'll have done it in a way that will last the rest of your life!

- **Present Tense.** Make sure you write your affirmations in the present tense. "I will lose weight" puts your success perpetually in the future because of the word *will*. "I am losing weight" puts your success where you want it: in the now.
- **Positive.** The subconscious mind doesn't register words like *no* and *not*. "I do not like cookies anymore" turns into "I do like cookies anymore" to the subconscious. Rather than stating what you don't want, state what you *do* want: "**I am toned**," versus "I am not fat"; "**I am happy**," versus "I am not sad"; "**I am employed**," versus "I am not unemployed anymore"; "**I am relaxed**," versus "I will become relaxed." Always go with the examples in bold, the ones that focus on what you want.
- **Concise and Easy to Memorize.** If your hypno-affirmations are so long that you can't memorize them, they won't be much good to you when you get to the step in self-hypnosis where you need to repeat it twenty-one times with your eyes closed. Concise hypno-affirmations are potent and more effective than a long-winded sentence.
- **One Topic at a Time.** If you're working on weight loss, just work on weight loss. Hold off on sleep, nail biting, and the rest until you've experienced the results you desire in weight loss. Otherwise

your subconscious will experience a system overload of sorts, and that will water down results across the board. For example, imagine you're watching a movie and are enthralled in the story line. The rest of the world melts away. You're not thinking about doing your taxes or emails you have to respond to; you're 100 percent in the movie. That's what happens when you focus on one topic at a time during hypnosis. If you attempt to work on weight loss and nail biting in the same hypnosis session, it would be like you watching a movie while texting back and forth with your friends. You'll miss key things that happen in the plot, and the texts will have spelling mistakes because you'll keep looking up at the screen. Both experiences will be diminished. Stick with one topic at a time, give it your all, and you'll experience lasting transformation much faster.

Why do I begin self-hypnosis with noticing my current stress level?

Knowing where you're starting on the stress scale helps you to gauge how much you've relaxed by the end of the practice. I've noticed that about half my clients will relax 50 percent or more during their first self-hypnosis process, about a quarter will relax more than 50 percent, and the other quarter will relax less than 50 percent.

25% of clients	Relax **more** than 50% with one round of self-hypnosis
50% of clients	Relax by 50% with one round of self-hypnosis
25% of clients	Relax **less** than 50% with one round of self-hypnosis and need two to three rounds to achieve optimal relaxation (any number below 5 on the stress scale is optimal)

Wherever you land on the scale after your first round of practice, know that you will relax significantly more with your second round. Go back and practice two rounds of self-hypnosis right now, back-to-back, to see what I mean!

Why do I lift the book up and memorize the hypno-affirmations on a diagonal before placing the book back down?

Have you ever noticed yourself becoming tired after staring at a computer screen for hours? It's not like you were chopping wood or doing anything physically taxing for hours. You were sitting and typing. So why the exhaustion? The light from the screen fatigues the eyes, and when the eyes become tired, it sets off a chain reaction for the entire body to relax deeply. In fact, this is why the silly swinging watch was a staple in early hypnosis; it tired clients' eyes and gave them something to focus on. Reading at an upward angle has a similar effect. Your eyes tire more quickly when you look up for an extended period, which sends a message to your body to relax. That being said, you want to be relaxed, not exhausted, so you only lift up the book for the time it takes to memorize the hypno-affirmation. Then you place the book back down and rest your hands comfortably in your lap.

Why do I imagine a color I love flowing in through the top of my head, all the way through my body?

Oftentimes, when you love a color, it features throughout your wardrobe, on the walls of your home, in trinkets throughout your office, even in the jewelry and artwork that you buy. By continually running the color you love through your body, it not only calms you but also conditions you to subconsciously feel calm every time you see that color throughout your day. You can change the color every time you practice this self-hypnosis process, or you can use the same color each time. I tend to find that blue is the most widely used, but any color or shade is perfect and correct.

Why do I count down from ten to one, saying "I am going deeper and deeper" after each number?

This is a wonderful, simple way to instruct the body and mind to relax. The key is to go slooooooowly. However slowly you went your first time practicing, go twice as slow next time and you'll experience even better results.

Why do I repeat the hypno-affirmation twenty-one times?

Despite its common occurrence in the world of personal development, twenty-one is not a *magical* number as far as building a new habit goes.[24] It is, however, just long enough that you'll get in a solid number of repetitions without taking so long that you'd skip self-hypnosis practice because of the investment of time required. If you're busy one day and can only repeat your hypno-affirmation ten times, or even three times, that's fine. A shorter practice is much better than no practice at all. Hypnosis is a process of conditioning.

---

24 James Clear, "How Long Does It Take to Form a New Habit?," HuffPost, May 29, 2015, www.huffpost.com/entry/form-new-habits_b_7346170.

A shorter conditioning session is infinitely more effective than no conditioning session, especially when it comes to weight loss.

Why is conditioning especially important for weight loss?

When someone stops smoking, everything gets thrown away: the cigarettes, the lighters, the ashtrays. That person is now a non-smoker. Nonsmokers don't walk around with an unlit cigarette hanging out of their lips just to see if they'll smoke it. The old habit is wiped out of one's life, and the temptations are removed. Weight loss is a little different. We still have to eat! We're never going to wipe food out of our lives. For this reason, practicing self-hypnosis right before each of your meals is an effective way to strengthen new pathways in the brain and to make sure that each meal will propel you further toward your weight loss goals.

Why do I visualize the desired outcome?

When you visualize the results you desire, you stimulate the part of the brain that is activated when you physically take that action. For example, visualizing or imagining that your body is slimmer or more toned—that you're fitting into certain clothes, that you feel energized, that your mind feels clear and happy, or that you're climbing a mountain or riding a bike or dancing a tango—creates a neural framework for you to not only **believe** these changes are possible for you but to cerebrally experience that they have in fact already taken place.

An example involving a group of university basket-ball players proves the power of visualizing while in hypnosis. In the study, one group of players was hypnotized while the other group was exposed to a variety of muscle relaxation techniques. According to the researcher,

> Results showed the hypnosis group scored significantly better (p < .05) than the relaxation group on dribbling scores, defensive scores and three-point shooting scores at post-intervention. The hypnosis group also scored significantly better (p < .05) at post-intervention than at pre-intervention on dribbling scores, defensive scores and speed shooting scores.[25]

Taking the time to visualize eating the way you want to eat, moving the way you want to move, feeling the way you want to feel, looking the way you want to look, will not only expedite your progress; it is a key factor in why you **will** succeed with your weight loss goals. If you had any lingering doubts—perhaps you're thinking, "I've tried everything, and nothing has worked"—take a nice, deep letting-go breath now and realize that unless you practiced daily visualization while in hypnosis, you not only haven't tried everything—you haven't tried the one thing that works! But from here on out, you will, and I'm so excited for you!

Why do I journal and track my sessions?

Without measurable data, your success will have to rely on your emotions or your willpower. Both of these will fail all of us more

25 Brian L. Vasquez, "The Effects of Hypnosis on Flow and in the Performance Enhancement of Basketball Skills" (PhD diss., Washington State University, College of Education, 2005), https://bscw.rediris.es/pub/bscw.cgi/d4434912/ Vasquez-Effects_hypnosis_flow_basketball_skills.pdf.

than we care to admit. But data is black and white—it's not emotional. You see where you're moving forward, where you're stalled, you see if there have been any steps in a direction you don't want, and then you can clearly and unemotionally make a decision about what to do next. That's why I have included journal pages to support your ongoing success. (You'll learn more about how to use them in the next chapter.) I'm excited for you to journal and track your sessions every day. If you choose to, you'll also be able to share your data with our online community (www.CloseYourEyesLose-Weight.com) so we can cheer you on!

Homework

A. Visit www.CloseYourEyesLoseWeight.com to listen to chapter two's hypnosis recording: "Mastering the Practice of Self-Hypnosis."

B. Every day, practice self-hypnosis three times (at breakfast, lunch, and dinnertime) using the hypno-affirmation "I am safe, I am calm. I choose to be here."

- - - - - - - - - - - - - - - -

Congratulations! You now know how to hypnotize yourself. You are ready to move on to chapter three, "Prepping for Your 90-Day Journey." You will learn how to get and remain motivated for a **lifetime of helpful choices**, as well as a **foolproof meal prep** process that will support you in eating well all week, without feeling overwhelmed. Let's get to it!

CHAPTER 3

. . . .

Prepping for Your 90-Day Journey

n this chapter you're going to prepare for your ninety-day journey by learning a number of skills:

- A new way to prep meals in advance so it's easier for you to stay on track with helpful eating throughout the week—no massive batches of brown rice included!
- How to create a new habit
- How to get and stay motivated (and how motivation is different from willpower)
- How to be on high alert for any potential pitfalls that could get in your way
- How to fill out the intake form that you will use as a benchmark for the next twelve weeks

Let's get started!

Meal Prep

For many of my clients, meal planning is on the top of their list of complaints before we begin our work together. Beth writes, "Meal planning is a huge struggle for me. I hate being decisive and feel bad if I make my boyfriend eat the same thing all the time, even though he wouldn't mind that in the least, so I tend to freeze up and eat like a toddler."

Let's break down the above:

- Meal planning is a huge struggle
- You're indecisive about what to make
- You don't want to subject those you cook for to the same few meals over and over
- So you do nothing and end up eating cheese sticks

Does this sound like you? You're not alone. In my experience, about 75 percent of the population does the same thing. If, however, you're a foodie who spends hours blissfully cooking every day, meal prep likely isn't a challenge for you. You can skip the rest of this section and move on to Willpower Versus Motivation.

The way I help my clients with meal prep is by teaching them to *automate* as much of the process as possible. There is a reason why John D. Rockefeller, Steve Jobs, Mark Zuckerberg, and other visionaries have been known to wear the same outfit every day; making decisions is mentally expensive. To have as much brainpower available as possible, many industry leaders opt to remove as much unnecessary decision making from their days as possible.

By automating your meal prep, you will stack the deck for success so you will have nourishing, helpful foods at the ready.

At the same time, if we make the meals too repetitive, the chances of you sticking with it for any length of time are slim. While common meal prepping advice includes making massive batches of food on Sunday evenings, that only works for those people who don't mind eating similar, if not identical, meals every day of the week. Perhaps my husband loves routine because he grew up eating rice and beans at every meal every single day of his life in Brazil. If you're the same way, more power to you! It's going to be even easier for you to automate your nourishing meals. But if your palate gets sick of the same thing pretty quickly, I find that cooking **one day ahead** increases meal prep success tenfold. The only thing you do on Sunday night is buy the food and make tomorrow's (Monday's) meals. That's it.

After a long and tiring day, having to make the meal you're *about* to eat can lend itself to giving up on the helpful option and choosing something quick, which is typically not helpful toward your weight loss goals. Instead, eat today's meals (made yesterday) and use the energy from that meal to spend twenty minutes making *tomorrow's* meals. The proactivity of this and the small amount of time required will motivate you to keep going, day after day. For this to work, you don't prep when you're hangry (hungry + angry) and you don't prep food you don't want to eat. This twenty-eight-day plan allows for variety, simplicity, and automation!

I know, I know. I can already hear you exclaim, "Grace, TWENTY-EIGHT meals?! That is way too many!" Take a nice, deep letting-go breath, my friend! A breakfast could be cereal with hemp milk (one meal down). A snack could be apple slices with cashew butter (two meals down). These are supposed to be **simple**. In the bonus resources online, you'll find a sample menu written by Jovanka Ciares, nutrition educator, wellness coach, and registered herbalist. Feel free to use it as is (plant-based) or adjust it to suit your dietary preferences. We've also broken the twenty-eight meals down into an easy shopping list for you. Find it at www.CloseYourEyesLoseWeight.com.

> Pro Tip: When making your meal plan, you can also use the recording in chapter six to make your meal plan based on your intuition.

You don't have to eat the same exact thing every day, but you can use the same meal plan every week, which is a huge plus if you love automating your life. Here's how you do it:

1. Make a list of twenty-eight healthy, helpful meals you love and that are easy to make. These include seven breakfasts, seven lunches, seven snacks, and seven dinners.
2. Visit www.CloseYourEyesLoseWeight.com to watch the how-to video. You'll also receive a fancy spreadsheet that will help you organize all the ingredients needed to make those twenty-eight simple meals. This will help you
   a) save money by only buying what you need;
   b) simplify your shopping; and
   c) make this repeatable each week (automation—woot!).
3. On Sundays, using your fancy spreadsheet, order or shop for all the food you'll need for the rest of the week.
4. For the rest of the week, only make *tomorrow's* meals today.

• • • • • • • • • • • • • • • •

Willpower Versus Motivation

Willpower (noun): control exerted to do something or restrain impulses.
Motivation (noun): the general desire or willingness of someone to do something.

"Grace, I need your help, but I don't know if it will work because I have no willpower." I've heard it a million times. If you're concerned about willpower, you can take a nice, deep letting-go breath and relax now.

The weight loss solution you're looking for is found in consistency and subconscious conditioning, not solely in willpower. In fact, even if you had all the willpower in the world, but your subconscious mind wanted something different from what your willpower wanted, willpower would lose every time.

Freud described the mind as an iceberg, with the conscious mind making up the part we see above the water (10 percent) and the subconscious mind taking up the entire mass beneath the surface (90 percent).

Willpower lives in the conscious mind, and as the conscious mind is only 10 percent of the equation that makes up who we are and why we do what we do, willpower alone can't be counted on to achieve one's weight loss goals. All it takes is one bad day, and willpower goes right out the window. Willpower isn't reliable enough to get us where we desire to go. You have to generate enough energy to rewire your subconscious while you make new conscious choices at the same time. With the help of hypnosis, this process will likely be more streamlined and effective than anything else you've tried before.

Willpower is about *controlling* impulses. Over time, hypnosis *removes* unhelpful impulses so there's nothing you'll need to try to control. Motivation, however, you need from beginning to end because motivation is the *desire* to keep going. Remember from page 27, hypnosis is not mind control and you must have a high level of *desire* to experience the result for the hypnosis to be effective. In this next section I will provide you the information necessary to keep your motivation high for the next twelve weeks, and beyond!

How to Get and Stay Motivated

In answer to the question "What were your greatest weight loss challenges in the past?" one Grace Spacer shared, "After the initial excitement of starting something new fades, I find that it is hard to stay motivated or keep up that level of excitement." Another responded, "Me, too! Busy life creates the opportunity to 'fall back' into old patterns."

The dreaded "old patterns" and "fading of initial excitement" are the downfall of so many worthy pursuits. The forces stopping you from creating *new* patterns and cultivating *sustained* excitement about a new endeavor are much more insidious than you might have imagined. What you're up against is called Resistance.

The opposite of motivation is Resistance, with a capital *R*. I first learned about it from Steven Pressfield. His short and engaging *The War of Art* is, in my opinion, a must read. In the book, Pressfield explains that any endeavor worth undertaking will be met with Resistance. Resistance wants to stop you from becoming your best self, it wants to stop you from being seen, and it wants to stop you from being better than you are now because to be better than you are now would require you to change your existing habits, and

Resistance positively hates that idea. Pressfield gives examples of the areas in life where we should expect Resistance to show up:

- Any diet or health regimen
- The pursuit of any calling in writing, painting, music, film, dance, or any creative art, however marginal or unconventional
- Any act that rejects immediate gratification in favor of long-term growth, health, or integrity
- Any act that derives from our higher nature instead of our lower[26]

Luckily, hypnosis helps overcome a tremendous amount of Resistance simply by virtue of aligning your subconscious beliefs with your conscious goals. However, conditioning your subconscious does take some time. In the interim it is important for you to be able to identify Resistance and defeat it. That might sound dramatic, but think about how many people you know who hate their bodies and eat things they don't want to eat and behave in ways they don't want to behave. Resistance's batting average is high. You cannot let it win any longer.

Put another way, Resistance is a lack of motivation to do something you wanted to do. It is also a clear sign that the subconscious is reverting to its old habits in an effort to *conserve energy*. It takes a tremendous amount of energy to change your ways. We want everything to be easy, we want what we want instantly, we hate the idea of having to work hard for what we want. But repetition, commitment, and perseverance are the keys that unlock anything worth achieving.

---

26 Steven Pressfield, *The War of Art* (New York: Black Irish Entertainment, 2002), 5–6.

You desire to lose weight and love the body you have.

Do you know what it takes to lose weight and love the body you have?

Are you committed and willing to do what it takes to lose weight and love the body you have?

Anytime the answer to that question is no . . .

You're not being lazy.

It's not a sign that you're weak.

You haven't given up.

You are facing Resistance!

Resistance is a real force that only wants you to do what you're already doing. Resistance doesn't want you to do what it takes to get the result you want, because that would require you to change—a lot! Change is Resistance's worst enemy.

"To defeat Resistance and get the results I want, I have to make <u>motivation</u> a HABIT."

Again, reread that last sentence three times with a nice, deep letting-go breath in between each round.

All human beings are programmed to create habitual behaviors because habits run automatically. Anything that runs automatically is energy efficient, and the body always wants to conserve energy in case it has to run away and protect itself.

What you must do is create *beneficial, helpful* habits that still run in the background and are *good* for you. So the initial motivation you experience, the initial desire to change, fueled by an upcoming high school reunion, or a health scare, or an inspiring Will Smith Instagram clip or movie, charges you with energy, enough energy to take a new action.

And maybe that new action lasts a few days, but inevitably, without that same reunion or health scare fueling us, we lose the *motivation*, the *energy* required to make a different choice. How do you make that willingness, that energy, last?

You program your *subconscious* mind to get motivated and *stay* motivated.

Why are drill sergeants always screaming at privates to do more push-ups? They don't lean over and whisper, "Oh, excuse me, would you mind doing more physical exercise than you ever have before, until your muscles convulse and you throw up to prove to me how badly you want to be a SEAL?"

No, they SCREAM at them because that adrenaline creates energy, and energy is required to get and stay motivated. New actions are energetically expensive, so you have to learn how to continually renew and fill up your energy bank account. If you find yourself falling off your plans or losing motivation, you've lost the energy required to take an action that is different from your habitual action.

Think of people running a marathon. The friends and family on the sidelines are not sitting down in chairs, quietly clapping, mouthing "good job, please continue." The people on the sidelines are jumping up and down, screaming, holding signs, giving high fives. They are transferring additional energy into the runners by being energetic themselves. When a joke falls flat, a comedian will say, "Tough crowd." Why is that? The audience is giving no *energy* to the comedian, and it starts to feel like an uphill battle to perform. You'll hear performers describe a fabulous crowd, by contrast, as "electric."

You must be *electric*. A conduit of actual energy. There is no shame, no guilt, no failing, simply energy—a lack thereof, a steady amount, or a surge of it. To desire a new result, to desire doing what it takes to make a new choice and then making that new choice, you need a *surge* of energy.

Do you see how looking at it this way makes it so clear? All the shame is allowed to leave your system now. Take a deep breath and watch it go. Bye-bye, shame! There is no "I'm a failure," "I'm so weak," "It's never going to happen for me," "I don't want it enough," "I'll always be like this." NO! It's a matter of getting curious: "Huh, I clearly need more energy right now so I can cultivate the motivation required to take an action that is different from the habitual action programmed in my brain. What's one way I can cultivate more energy right now?" That's a great question and great questions elicit great answers. Practice asking that out loud right now:

"What's one way I can cultivate more energy right now?"

Ask this in place of "What's wrong with me?" every single time Resistance tries to get you to think it. "Cancel, cancel!" that thought. "Cancel, cancel!" it and replace it with "What's one way I can cultivate more energy right now?" (Return to page 15 for a refresher on how to use the "Cancel, cancel!" technique.)

Here are some things I want you to do to cultivate more energy right now:

1. Listen to your favorite pump-up musical anthem.

> A few of my clients' favorite pump-up anthems are "Don't Hurt Yourself" by Beyoncé and "Lose Yourself" by Eminem. "Happy" by Pharrell Williams is a good PG-rated choice.

2. Do ten jumping jacks (just ten—you don't get extra points for doing more right now, since this has to be a quick process) or roll up onto your toes, reach your arms up over your head toward the ceiling, come back down onto flat feet, and repeat this stretch nine more times.

3. Then sit back, close your eyes, and listen to the chapter three recording found at www. CloseYourEyesLoseWeight.com.

Now that you're done, how do you feel? More energy? Enough energy to make a new, better, healthier choice? Awesome. Let's get this down on paper so you can remember it when you need it next:

Write down how you feel right now and, most importantly, write yourself a call to action for you to come back here and do this EXACT sequence anytime Resistance pops up in your life.

If you find yourself falling off course at any point over the next ninety days, no problem! Everyone falls off the bike when first learning to ride. You now know what to do to get back on and pedal even further:

- Reject self-sabotage's desire to reach for shame, guilt, and ugly thoughts because they only dig the hole deeper. Reject those ideas outright. This is black and white and unemotional. It's Resistance. Everyone has it, but you won't let it win.
- You recognize Resistance has swung by for a visit.
- You recognize you require a surge of energy so you can get motivated.
- Once you're back to being motivated, it's much easier for you to make the right choice and drive Resistance out of town.
- Rinse, wash, repeat. Reject shame, cultivate energy, reinstate motivation, make the right choice.

For the rest of this ninety-day journey (and for the rest of your life), any time you "don't want to do it" or find yourself making an unhelpful choice or giving into lame-o excuses, say its name out loud: "Resistance . . . I see you!" You now have so many ways you can defeat Resistance in that moment. Come back to this chapter, reread it, cultivate energy, listen to the chapter three hypnosis recording provided at www.CloseYourEyesLoseWeight.com, practice this week's self-hypnosis, document your experiences in your journal pages, and get back to work because you are worth it!

Learning a New Habit

Think about what it was like to learn to drive a car. Even for those of us who learned to drive in an automatic car, but especially for those of you who learned to drive a manual car, it is awkward at first. It was clunky, jarring, literally stop-and-go, back and forth, stopping short, trying to check all the mirrors and look where you have to go while not stalling out. It was not comfortable, and it was *not* automatic. This is what learning a brand-new habit is always like. When you learn the habit in the subconscious mind, it becomes an automatic habit much faster than when attempting to learn it only consciously. (Parents with kids about to get their permits: remember this and check out our "Learning to Drive" Grace Space hypnosis recording!) But even with the help of hypnosis, learning a new habit is still going to be a bit clunky at first. Just keep going.

A few additional and important final no-no's when prepping for your ninety-day journey and you'll be on your way.

Avoid the following:

- Waiting until you're extremely hungry. Plan to avoid this—eat before the major hunger pains arise to limit overeating or scarfing down food.
- Standing in front of the pantry or fridge while hungry, thinking, "Hmm, what should I have?" Plan to

avoid this—already know what you're going to eat in advance and make it the day before. My toddler has taught me an important lesson—if he sees a healthier choice next to an unhealthy but "yummier" food, he goes for what is tastier in the short term, every time. But if I only offer him one option, the healthy option, he happily munches away without complaint. You want to avoid unhelpful options altogether.

- Food shopping on a whim while hungry. Plan to avoid this—only ever shop for food when you're not hungry and when you have a plan of what ingredients you need to buy for your week's worth of meals.
- Hitting a drive-through with lots of tempting, unhelpful food options because you only have five minutes to eat. Plan to avoid this—have healthy snacks on you at all times so if you forget your lunch box or your schedule runs away from you, you're going into your bag for a banana or a handful of nuts instead of ordering a batch of deep-fried potatoes.

The most important thing is that you remove these from your experience entirely:

- Shame
- Guilt
- "I'm failing."
- "What's wrong with me?"

"Cancel, cancel!" all those old, unhelpful thoughts. Read the following passage out loud and copy it down in your own handwriting in the space provided. Then read it to yourself every time you need a pick-me-up:

I promise to get curious. I promise to stay neutral. When I see the data heading in an unhelpful direction, it lets me know which areas would benefit from additional conditioning. That's all. That area simply needs more conditioning. I adjust my daily hypnosis practices to give those areas more attention. I continue to track the data and look forward to progressing in all areas over time. I am learning. I am doing great. I am proud of myself. This is fun!

_____

_____

_____

_____

_____

_____

_____

_____

_____

_____

_____

_____

_____

_____

_____
_____
_____
_____
_____
_____
_____
_____
_____
_____
_____
_____

Signature _____

Date _____

Now you are ready for your official intake form.

Intake Form

(A) Weight   (B) Measurements   (C) How You Feel in Your Clothes   (D) Energy Level

If you're tracking your weight or measurements, record your starting numbers below. If you choose to track how your clothes fit or your energy level, indicate how you currently feel on a scale of 1 to 5, 1 as the worst and 5 as the best.

INTAKE	Weight		Measurements		How Do You Feel in Your Clothes?	What's Your Energy Level?
	Weight at start date:	Neck:		Waist:		
		Chest:		Hips:	1 2 3 4 5	1 2 3 4 5
	90-day weight goal:	(L) Arm		(L) Thigh:		
		(R) Arm		(R) Thigh:		

What is your natural weight?

What weight do you know you can easily achieve?

Why do you want to lose weight?

Why don't you want to lose weight?

When do you eat?

Where do you eat?

Why do you eat?

What foods do you have trouble with (salty/sweets/carbs/etc.)?

What are some alternatives to eating, if you're simply bored?

What are some alternative foods?

Are large portions a problem?

Are second helpings a problem?

Do you exercise?

Have you dieted?

Close your eyes. Can you imagine (desired outcome)?

It's likely you received some powerful and new insights while filling out the above. Take note as you work your way through the recordings I've made for you each week where your **subconscious** ideas differ from your what your conscious mind wrote above. As a bonus, if you ever choose to work with one of our Grace Space hypnotherapists, they will ask you the same questions above, so you'll be a step ahead in being able to share this information with them during your first session (visit www.CloseYourEyesLoseWeight.com for more information). It will also be fascinating and rewarding for you to return to your intake form after these first ninety days are complete—you'll see how much you've transformed!

Homework

A. Practice self-hypnosis three times a day, every day this week (right before breakfast, lunch, and dinner). Turn to page 20 for a reminder of how to do self-hypnosis or head to www.CloseYourEyesLoseWeight.com to follow along with a tutorial video.

B. Listen to the "Prep Week—Motivation" hypnosis recording every day for the next week here: www.CloseYourEyesLoseWeight.com.

C. Use your journal pages daily to stay motivated, log your progress, and determine which pick-me-up hypno-affirmations you'll benefit from most this week.

Hypno-affirmations—Motivation

- I seek out ways to cultivate energy.
- By cultivating energy, I easily stay motivated.
- I am worthy and deserving of sticking with this.
- I am worthy of doing what it takes to be healthy.
- I recognize Resistance and do what it takes to defeat it!
- I make tomorrow's meals today so I am healthy every day.

· · · · · · · · · · · · · · · ·

You've got meal prep under control, you've got the necessary **tools** to **cultivate the energy** required to get and stay **motivated**. It's time to move on! In the next chapter you'll be shocked to learn what happens when your subconscious learns how to eat properly, how to hydrate properly, how to stop eating when you're full, and more. Do ten jumping jacks or toe roll-ups (just ten!) to get even more excited about what's coming next, then turn the page.

PART II

. . . .

Weeks 1–4

Progress Tracker

POUNDS LOST

Starting Weight _____

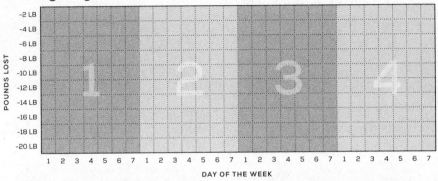

DAY OF THE WEEK

HOW DO YOU FEEL IN YOUR CLOTHES ?

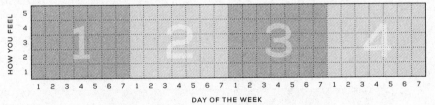

DAY OF THE WEEK

WHAT'S YOUR ENERGY LEVEL?

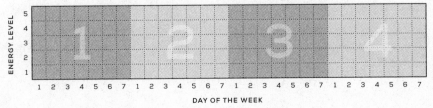

DAY OF THE WEEK

Starting Waist Measurement _____

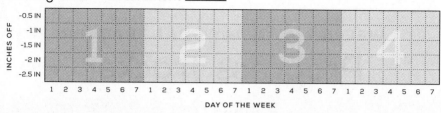

Starting Thigh (L) Measurement _____

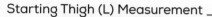
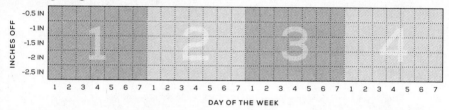

Starting Thigh (R) Measurement _____

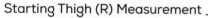
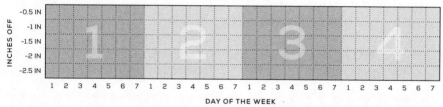

Starting Neck Measurement _____

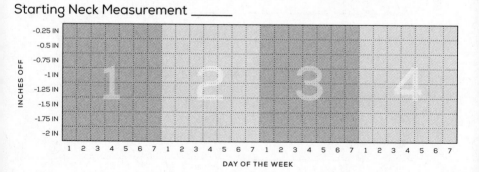

Starting Hip Measurement _____

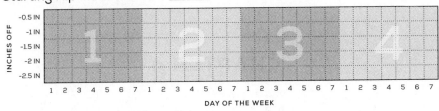

Starting Arm (L) Measurement _____

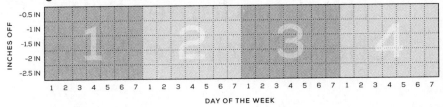

Starting Arm (R) Measurement _____

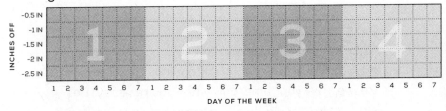

Starting Chest Measurement _____

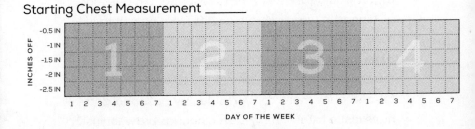

CHAPTER 4

· · · · · · · · · · · · · · · ·

Week 1–
The Fundamentals:
Chew, Hydrate, Stop!

"Grace is going to tell you to chew, a lot. At first my husband kept teasing me by saying, 'By all means, Bessie, take your time, only when you're ready.' Bessie . . . as in the cow, because I was chewing for so long that it would take me ages to respond to a question at dinner! It was such a big shift from how quickly I used to eat. But I lost twenty-two pounds, and it's been so easy to keep it off that my entire family is on the chewing train now. Dinner is a lot more thoughtful and a lot more comfortable. My husband and I have lost a total of forty-seven pounds between us!" –Latisha T., Camden, New Jersey

Start your engines! You've completed all the necessary preparations, and now it's time to officially begin your twelve-week weight loss journey!

Ah, the fundamentals. These puppies are Weight Loss 101. The building blocks upon which you will build your success. Don't let these steps deceive you. They may sound simple, but it's going to take commitment for you to condition these new behaviors into your subconscious mind. Cultivate some energy using the techniques you learned in the previous chapter, and dive in!

Chew

You are going to spend a good deal of time teaching your subconscious the importance of chewing. It's incredible how many challenges you can overcome by chewing correctly. I'm going to be a tad graphic in this chapter **on purpose**. You want to create negative subconscious associations with the things you don't want to do anymore. "Negative associations" don't mean failure or guilt—remember to always "Cancel, cancel!" those feelings. In this context, negative is simply the opposite of positive—what is not good for you versus what is good for you.

When you swallow big, thick chunks of food, they sit and rot in your stomach. You don't realize you're full when you eat too quickly. Your body has to work so hard to digest those massive chunks of food that it steals energy away from cognitive and healing functions.

To solve this, you will condition yourself to chew all your food until only liquid remains. You are turning your delicious meals into a juice so only liquid is hitting your stomach. This means you will begin to eat more slowly (it takes a while to chew until only liquid remains!), you will stop eating sooner (by eating slower, your body has a chance to get the signal that you're satisfied—more on this in a moment), and your body can utilize the nutrients from the food you're eating because you've already done most of the work. When the digestive system doesn't have to work so hard to break down massive chunks of rotting food, there is energy left over. That energy is used by your brain to think and your body to function and heal. In fact, Dr. Harald Stossier, director of a prestigious medi-clinic in Austria, has said, "A well-chewed burger is better for your waistline than a badly chewed salad."[27]

In an article entitled "Why Chewing Your Food Can Change Your Life," Dr. Alejandra Carrasco writes about why chewing is so important:

1. It triggers digestion.
2. It promotes growth and repair in the body.
3. It's a foundation for disease prevention.[28]

Do you find that after a meal it's common for you to feel exhausted? It could be because all your surplus energy is now being spent on breaking down food. Randy Santel sheds light on this in the context of eating competitions:

All of your body's energy is being used by your digestive system—your digestive organs, especially your large and

---

27 Laura Holland, "Chew on This: 7 Reasons Not to Gobble Up Your Food," *National*, December 8, 2014, www.thenational.ae/lifestyle/food/chew-on-this-7 -reasons-not-to-gobble-up-your-food-1.456600.
28 Alejandra Carrasco, "Why Chewing Your Food Can Change Your Life," mindbodygreen, accessed November 4, 2019, www.mindbodygreen.com/0-7775 /why-chewing-your-food-can-change-your-life.html.

small intestines, require a large amount of energy to work effectively and function properly. After a big . . . meal, your body is going crazy trying to digest and process the thousands of calories you just quickly consumed. To do this, your brain diverts most of your body's energy and focus toward digestion . . . This is why you feel fatigued . . . Your body is exhausting all of its energy trying to digest the big meal.[29]

Could you imagine what it would be like to enjoy a meal and feel energized afterward? To feel light instead of heavy? To never be bloated again?! This is what chewing every bite until only liquid remains can do for you. An article in the *National* points out several reasons why chewing your food slowly is one of the most powerful things you can do for better health:

Undigested food takes more space in your stomach than digested food and creates bloating, thus slowing down the entire digestive process . . . Chewing slowly also helps increase the alkalinity of the food, which is extremely important. Many people suffer from acid reflux, heart burn, and indigestion, and while some foods—even if chewed well—trigger these problems, it is important to note that the longer you chew, the less acid is formed.[30]

I'm going to be a real stickler about this chewing thing, so let's get all the objections (read: Resistance!) I'm used to hearing out of the way:

---

29 Randy Santel, "Why Your Body Feels Tired After Eating a Lot," Food Challenges, June 14, 2018, www.foodchallenges.com/after-the-challenge/why-your-body-feels-tired-after-eating/.
30 Holland, "Chew on This."

"It takes a while to chew my food until only liquid remains!"
Yes. Yes, it does . . . And that is the point. Note that you're not to
chew every bite ten or a hundred times. Every bite will be different
depending on what you're eating. Regardless of how long it takes,
you must chew it until only liquid remains. Imagine someone rip-
ping off a massive bite of turkey club, chomping down three times,
swallowing the huge glob of food with a massive gulp so they can
continue talking, bits of food flying out of the mouth, burps escap-
ing . . . Hey, I told you I was going to get graphic on purpose! How
are those negative associations coming along?

Now, take a nice, deep letting-go breath and instead imagine
someone taking a comfortably sized bite and slowly, thoughtfully
chewing until only liquid remains, which makes it easy to swallow,
and *then* speaking. Imagine how each of their bodies feels. Decide
which actions you'd like to take not by what you've always done
or by what society or culture dictates but by deciding how you
would like to *feel* and which set of actions will support that feeling.
Remember, if your meal takes longer, you'll feel better.

"My jaw hurts." That's likely because you have tiny baby jaw
muscles that were never trained to chew. Like any muscle, they'll
get stronger with practice. Chewing until only liquid remains will
become comfortable so long as you stick with it. The hypnosis
recording for this chapter will help you do just that.

**"It's hard to have a conversation over a meal if I'm chew-
ing until only liquid remains."** Listen more, talk less. Enjoy your
food more, scarf way less (ideally, scarf never). Chew more, eat less.
Your chewing could improve the eating pace for everyone you're
with, and you'll **taste** your food. The bonus is, by listening more
while you chew, you simultaneously improve all your relationships!
Monks don't eat and talk; they eat or talk. This is called "mindful
eating." There's no way to be mindful about your eating if you can't

taste what's in your mouth. Slow down, chew, chew, chew, chew, chew, chew.

"But, Grace, it's been a few days and I'm still not chewing like a pro yet." Let's be honest. Most people have been scarfing down their food without chewing it for their entire lives. Cut yourself some slack! You're learning something brand new here. The first step is awareness—becoming aware of how quickly you were eating, how big those unchewed chunks were as they sat there in your stomach, causing gas and bloating. Causing exhaustion as your body worked overtime to *try* to squeeze a few nutrients from those rotting globs. That awareness is such a gift. It's such a transformation. It's brand new. Take a nice, deep letting-go breath and release any judgment. Stick with it; it takes time to recondition the subconscious mind, but happily, with hypnosis, it takes a lot less time than any other method.

. . . .

Learning to chew and sticking with it until it becomes an automatic behavior will change your life forever.

The hypnosis recording at the end of this chapter will begin to program your subconscious mind to chew like a pro, but in the meantime, jump-start your new automatic behavior with a round of self-hypnosis and choose from the following hypno-affirmations:

- Every day in every way I chew my food more and more.
- I chew every bite until only liquid remains.
- The more I chew, the faster I lose weight.
- The more I chew, the sooner I'm satisfied.
- By chewing my food until only liquid remains, I lose weight and feel great.

Hydrate

In your weekly foundations hypnosis recording you will program your subconscious mind to drink one eight-ounce glass of water before every meal. It's simple, easy to remember, and you will lose more weight this way.

> Researchers from Virginia Tech compared weight loss between two groups of participants. One group was instructed to consume water before eating low-calorie meals, while the other ate low-calorie meals without increasing their water intake. The researchers found that over a twelve-week period, those who drank water before meals, three times a week, lost about five pounds more than those who did not.[31] Another 2010 study from Vanderbilt University found that water increases activity in the sympathetic nervous system, which causes your body to burn more calories. They also found that drinking three sixteen-ounce glasses of water a day increases calorie burning enough to help you drop five pounds in a year without making any other changes to your lifestyle.[32]

31 Elizabeth A. Dennis et al., "Water Consumption Increases Weight Loss During a Hypocaloric Diet Intervention in Middle-Aged and Older Adults," *Obesity (Silver Spring)* 18, no. 2 (2010), 300–307, www.ncbi.nlm.nih.gov/pmc/articles/PMC2859815/.
32 Vanderbilt University Medical Center, "Water's Unexpected Role in Blood Pressure Control," ScienceDaily, July 14, 2010, www.sciencedaily.com/releases/2010/07/100706150639.htm

In addition to a bonus five pounds of weight loss, there are many other reasons to increase your daily consumption of H_2O. The more water you drink, the less hungry you become. Often a "hunger pain" sensation is thirst. When dehydrated, we don't think as clearly, and the digestive system starts to slow down.

According to *Quench* by Dana Cohen and Gina Bria, hydration is not just beneficial, it is the essence of our health: "You are a body of water. In fact . . . approximately 65 percent of you is water. If you're not hydrated, everything else you do to stay healthy (exercising, eating right, stress management, sleep) is undercut."[33]

Sources of dehydration include salt-heavy foods, moisture-lacking processed foods, a diet lacking in greens and fruits, fluorescent lighting, dry heat, air-conditioning, electronic devices, immobility, and medications used to reduce pain, stiffness, allergies, or any chronic condition.[34] The authors share that chronic dehydration is a common health issue for residents of nursing homes, and it's easy to see why when reviewing the list of contributing factors above. But that's not all—the authors cite the *European Journal of Nutrition*, which states that some doctors think as many as 75 percent of Americans are chronically dehydrated![35]

In addition to drinking the right amount of water each day, Cohen and Bria share many tips to stay hydrated. Here are some favorites that I learned from *Quench*:

- Eat the top twelve hydrating veggies: cucumbers, romaine lettuce, celery, radishes, zucchini,

---

33 Dana Cohen and Gina Bria, *Quench* (New York: Hachette Books, 2018), x–xi.
34 Cohen and Bria, *Quench*, 2.
35 Giannis Arnaoutis et al., "The Effect of Hypohydration on Endothelial Function in Young, Healthy Adults," *European Journal of Nutrition* 56, no. 3 (2017): 1211–17, https://link.springer.com/article/10.1007%2Fs00394-016-1170-8.

tomatoes, peppers, cauliflower, spinach, broccoli, carrots, sprouts. Eat the top twelve hydrating fruits, which include star fruit, watermelon, strawberries, grapefruit, cantaloupe, pineapple, raspberries, blueberries, kiwi, apples, pears, and grapes.

- Instead of salting your food, salt your water with a pinch of sea salt, Celtic salt, rock salt, or Himalayan salt (never processed table salt) and you will have "a simple way to make sure you have the ideal electrolyte exchange to keep water balanced inside you."[36]

- Add one tablespoon of chia seeds to your water or smoothies.[37] Chia seeds help you to stay hydrated for longer periods. Similar to the ways in which desert communities stay hydrated by eating things like cactus, a plant that has incredible water-retaining capabilities, chia seeds expand when wet, so they help you retain more water for longer.

Bathroom Breaks

Despite all the benefits of hydration, one line of Resistance I often hear is, "I know I need to drink more water, but I hate getting up to go to the bathroom so often. Everyone in my office knows where I'm headed, and it's annoying, embarrassing, and breaks up my work flow." I feel you, but remember

---

36 Cohen and Bria, *Quench*, 68.
37 Cohen and Bria, *Quench*, 187.

that everyone is focused on themselves 99.99 percent of the time. It's unlikely your coworkers are tracking your bathroom breaks as much as you think they are. Are you tracking theirs? Probably not—I hope not, anyway! We're all focused on ourselves all day long, and yet we worry so much about what other people think. It's a terrible use of time. As far as breaking up work flow goes—a small break from one's desk or computer screen is a positive! "The key to losing weight with a desk job is to look for ways to move more and sit less."[38]

Your first way of overcoming this Resistance will be to repeat this mantra in your mind every time you get up to use the restroom: "This is great! I'm hydrated, cleansing my system, getting a quick break, AND losing weight. I'm so proud of myself!" Pretty soon you'll have reprogrammed your mind to feel gratitude rather than Resistance every time you take a sip.

In summary, staying hydrated is not only important for weight loss; it's important for your comprehensive health. The next fundamental for you to master is to stop eating when you're "satisfied."

---

38 Julia Guerra, "17 Tips for Staying Healthy While Working a Desk Job," Insider, January 29, 2019, www.insider.com/weight-loss-tips-for-people-who -work-a-lot-2018-11.

Stop When You Are Satisfied

As a child, were you told to eat everything on your plate "because people are starving in [fill in a foreign country]?" I was. And most of my clients were, too. This is a 1950s, post-Depression, post-WWII, outdated way of training us not to waste food. While it's wonderful to want to make a difference, eating all the food on our plates doesn't affect the hunger of anyone else. At the heart of the saying is a weird association between being a good person and eating all the food on one's plate; therefore, if one doesn't, it follows that one is a "bad" person.

To teach kids not to waste food, it is much more effective to *make* less food in the first place and to *put* less food on their plates. Yes, you'll need to chat with your Italian, Brazilian, Jewish, Greek, and [fill in your *love-is-often-expressed-through-food* heritage] grandparents about their propensity to scoop heaps of food onto unsuspecting plates and then become palpably hurt, shocked, or miffed when round three isn't consumed joyously. Scooping on heaps of food, forcing ourselves to eat it, and then praising ourselves when we've finished it all is a lame way of getting a "win" for the day. We want to be praised. We want that pat on the back when the plate is all clean. Here's a recipe for disaster:

Too much food cooked
+ too much food on plate
+ I'm a bad boy/girl if I don't finish my plate
+ I've accomplished something if my plate is clean
= very unhelpful if you'd like to lose weight.

We have to switch the reward. The reward, the prize, will now come from leaving food *on* your plate. Not a ton, but some. A clean plate now becomes the "failure," as far as the subconscious mind is concerned. Rather than racing toward the finish line of "Clean plate! Clean plate!" you're able to slow down and with each bite assess if you want the next one. The *goal* is to leave food **on** the plate.

> This is the winning recipe:
>
> Cook less food so massive helpings aren't an option
> + only take half of what you think you'll want
> + chew every bite until only liquid remains
> + only get more if you are still hungry after mindfully eating the first portion
> + stop eating when you are 90 percent satisfied
> + feeling you WIN when there is still some food on your plate
> = weight loss, feeling light, a lack of bloating, improved energy, and showing your body love.

Are your environmentally friendly Spidey senses shutting down this idea? I commend your principles! Let's review: make less food to start (save the planet), eat less food (save your health), leave some food on the plate to retrain your brain that *that* is the "win," and then save your leftovers or compost them! You don't have to toss the uneaten food into the bin. While "eat all the food on your plate because there are starving children in the world" doesn't change the world in any way, if you genuinely feel called to help fight hunger and make the world a better place,

consider making a donation to Action Against Hunger (www.
actionagainsthunger.org) or eating plant-based meals a few more
times each week. As CNN reported, "An assessment by the Food
and Agriculture Organization of the United Nations indicated the
contribution of the livestock sector to global greenhouse gas emissions exceeds that of transportation. It follows that . . . adopting
a plant-based diet is, therefore, one of the most powerful choices
an individual can make in mitigating environmental degradation
and depletion of Earth's natural resources."[39]

Another piece in HuffPost explains that "world leaders are set
to endorse a UN goal to eliminate hunger by 2030, but . . . diets
must feature less red meat, which consumes eleven times more
water and results in five times more climate-warming emissions
than chicken or pork, according to a 2014 study. The shift . . .
must apply to both wealthy and developing nations, where consumption of ecologically unfriendly foods is growing fastest." The
same article quotes biologist Colin Khoury: "Sustainable and
healthy diets will require a move towards a mostly plant-based
diet."[40] Now that you're armed with real ways to make a difference,
you can happily retrain your brain to leave a bit of food on your
plate with a clear conscience.

Feeling better already? Wait until you're through with the next
section. I wonder how much lighter you'll feel.

39 George C. Wang, "Go Vegan, Save the Planet," CNN, April 9, 2017, www.
cnn.com/2017/04/08/opinions/go-vegan-save-the-planet-wang/index.html.
40 Chris Arsenault, "Cutting Back on Meat Consumption Could Help End
Hunger by 2030: Experts," HuffPost, September 11, 2015, www.huffpost.com/
entry/cutting-back-on-meat-consumption-could-help-end-hunger-by-2030-ex-
perts_n_55f3424ee4b077ca094f27a5.

"I'm Satisfied" Versus "I'm Full"
Versus "I'm Stuffed"

At the end of a meal, my Brazilian husband says, "I'm satisfied." In Portuguese, *estou satisfeito* translates to "I'm satisfied" and is used instead of "I'm full," which to the Brazilian ear sounds pretty gross. And that's already a vast improvement over "I'm stuffed," which conjures images of a pig on a spit with an apple shoved in its lifeless mouth.

This cultural difference got me thinking. In the United States, we tend to believe that a "good meal" is when we leave "full" or "stuffed." When we take a step back, that does sound pretty gross and uncomfortable, doesn't it? What if we stopped eating when we were "satisfied" instead? Doesn't that sound a lot lighter and more comfortable?

With this week's hypnosis recording you're going to begin training yourself to stop eating when you're satisfied and remove "I'm full" and "I'm stuffed" from both your experience and your vocabulary. When you consume food in a helpful way, you stop eating as soon as you are satisfied. In fact, you stop eating as soon as you are 90 percent satisfied because that remaining 10 percent is typically satiated with time (the gut registering how much food it has had) or with hydration.

After a meal, your gut suppresses a hormone called ghrelin, which controls hunger, while also releasing fullness hormones.[41] These hormones tell your brain

41 Gavin A. Bewick, "Bowels Control Brain: Gut Hormones and Obesity," *Biochemia Medica* 22, no. 3 (2012): 283–97, www.ncbi.nlm.nih.gov/pubmed/23092061.

that you have eaten, reducing appetite, making you feel satisfied, and helping you stop eating. This process takes about twenty minutes, so slowing down gives your brain the time it needs to receive these signals.

What time should you stop eating at night?

Even well-chewed food can disturb your sleep. If you want to get rid of those dark circles under your eyes, have more energy, and feel more full of life, chew every bite until only liquid remains and stop eating at least two hours before you go to bed.

In summary, training your subconscious mind that the **helpful** way to eat includes chewing every bite until only liquid remains, drinking water before each meal, and eating slowly enough that your body has time to register when you are *satisfied* will set you free.

Remember, there's no shame allowed here. This is black and white: you're either eating in a helpful way that supports your weight loss or you're eating in an unhelpful way that supports weight gain or stagnation. You are programming your subconscious to choose helpful beliefs and actions so you can reach your goals faster.

Great job! I'm so excited for you to notice how good you feel when you commit to chewing every bite until only liquid remains, drinking a glass of water before every meal with a focus on staying hydrated throughout the day, and stopping eating when you are 90 percent satisfied.

Homework

A. Practice self-hypnosis three times a day, every day this week (right before breakfast, lunch, and dinner). Turn back to page 20 for a reminder of how to do self-hypnosis or head to www. CloseYourEyesLoseWeight.com to follow along with a tutorial video.

Week 1 Hypno-affirmations—Foundations (Chew, Hydrate, Stop)

- I chew every bite of food until only liquid remains.
- The more I chew, the more weight I lose.
- When I want the weight to go, I grab another glass of H_2O.
- I drink a glass of water before every meal.
- When I feel 90 percent satisfied, I stop eating.
- Every day in every way it's easier and easier to stop eating when I am almost satisfied.

B. Listen to the "Week 1—Foundations" hypnosis recording every day for the next week here: www. CloseYourEyesLoseWeight.com.

C. Use your journal pages daily to stay motivated, log your progress, and determine which pick-me-up hypno-affirmations you'll benefit from most.

Great job! Now that you've begun the process of mastering the fundamentals of weight loss, it's time to move on to a major detractor of weight loss success . . . limiting beliefs. You'll learn about dozens of subconscious limiting beliefs that have to go so weight loss success becomes inevitable.

WEEK 1 LOG

TRACK YOUR PROGRESS

TODAY

Weight	Measurements	How Do You Feel in Your Clothes?	What's Your Energy Level?
	Neck: Waist:		
	Chest: Hips:	1 2 3 4 5	1 2 3 4 5
	(L) Arm (L) Thigh:		
	(R) Arm (R) Thigh:		

Write down any negative thoughts, immediately cross them out, and replace them with a positive thought.

CANCEL-CANCEL BOX

[PRO TIP] Stay neutral. Get curious!

How Will You Conjure Up Additional Energy When Needed?

10 jumping jacks ___   Shout hypno-affirmations ___   Other ___

Water

8oz of water before breakfast ___   8oz of water before lunch ___   8oz of water before dinner ___

This Morning's Self-Hypnosis | Round 1: Week 1—Fundamentals

Time you start: _____   Starting Stress Level (0–10): _____   Ending Stress Level (0–10): _____

This Afternoon's Self-Hypnosis | Round 2: Week 1—Fundamentals

Time you start: _____   Starting Stress Level (0–10): _____   Ending Stress Level (0–10): _____

This Evening's Self-Hypnosis | Round 3: Week 1—Fundamentals

Time you start: _____   Starting Stress Level (0–10): _____   Ending Stress Level (0–10): _____

Listen to this week's assigned hypnotherapy recording (found at www.CloseYourEyesLoseWeight.com): ☐

Tomorrow's Meal Planning

Breakfast	Snack	Lunch	Snack	Dinner

Check here when tomorrow's meals have been made or ordered: ☐

Visit www.CloseYourEyesLoseWeight.com and share your wins with our community: ☐

WEEK 1 LOG

TRACK YOUR PROGRESS

TODAY

Weight	Measurements	How Do You Feel in Your Clothes?	What's Your Energy Level?
	Neck: Waist:		
	Chest: Hips:	1 2 3 4 5	1 2 3 4 5
	(L) Arm (L) Thigh:		
	(R) Arm (R) Thigh:		

Write down any negative thoughts, immediately cross them out, and replace them with a positive thought.

CANCEL-CANCEL BOX

[PRO TIP] Stay neutral. Get curious!

How Will You Conjure Up Additional Energy When Needed?

10 jumping jacks __   Shout hypno-affirmations __   Other __

Water

8oz of water before breakfast __   8oz of water before lunch __   8oz of water before dinner __

This Morning's Self-Hypnosis | Round 1: Week 1—Fundamentals

Time you start: _____   Starting Stress Level (0–10): _____   Ending Stress Level (0–10): _____

This Afternoon's Self-Hypnosis | Round 2: Week 1—Fundamentals

Time you start: _____   Starting Stress Level (0–10): _____   Ending Stress Level (0–10): _____

This Evening's Self-Hypnosis | Round 3: Week 1—Fundamentals

Time you start: _____   Starting Stress Level (0–10): _____   Ending Stress Level (0–10): _____

Listen to this week's assigned hypnotherapy recording (found at www.CloseYourEyesLoseWeight.com): ☐

Tomorrow's Meal Planning

Breakfast	Snack	Lunch	Snack	Dinner

Check here when tomorrow's meals have been made or ordered: ☐

Visit www.CloseYourEyesLoseWeight.com and share your wins with our community: ☐

WEEK 1 LOG

TRACK YOUR PROGRESS

TODAY

Weight	Measurements		How Do You Feel in Your Clothes?	What's Your Energy Level?
	Neck:	Waist:		
	Chest:	Hips:	1 2 3 4 5	1 2 3 4 5
	(L) Arm	(L) Thigh:		
	(R) Arm	(R) Thigh:		

Write down any negative thoughts, immediately cross them out, and replace them with a positive thought.

CANCEL-CANCEL BOX

[PRO TIP] Stay neutral. Get curious!

How Will You Conjure Up Additional Energy When Needed?

10 jumping jacks ___   Shout hypno-affirmations ___   Other ___

Water

8oz of water before breakfast ___   8oz of water before lunch ___   8oz of water before dinner ___

This Morning's Self-Hypnosis | Round 1: Week 1—Fundamentals

Time you start: _____   Starting Stress Level (0–10): _____   Ending Stress Level (0–10): _____

This Afternoon's Self-Hypnosis | Round 2: Week 1—Fundamentals

Time you start: _____   Starting Stress Level (0–10): _____   Ending Stress Level (0–10): _____

This Evening's Self-Hypnosis | Round 3: Week 1—Fundamentals

Time you start: _____   Starting Stress Level (0–10): _____   Ending Stress Level (0–10): _____

Listen to this week's assigned hypnotherapy recording (found at www.CloseYourEyesLoseWeight.com): ☐

Tomorrow's Meal Planning

Breakfast	Snack	Lunch	Snack	Dinner

Check here when tomorrow's meals have been made or ordered: ☐

Visit www.CloseYourEyesLoseWeight.com and share your wins with our community: ☐

TRACK YOUR PROGRESS

TODAY

Weight	Measurements	How Do You Feel in Your Clothes?	What's Your Energy Level?
	Neck: Waist:		
	Chest: Hips:	1 2 3 4 5	1 2 3 4 5
	(L) Arm (L) Thigh:		
	(R) Arm (R) Thigh:		

Write down any negative thoughts, immediately cross them out, and replace them with a positive thought.

CANCEL-CANCEL BOX

[PRO TIP] Stay neutral. Get curious!

How Will You Conjure Up Additional Energy When Needed?

10 jumping jacks ___   Shout hypno-affirmations ___   Other ___

Water

8oz of water before breakfast ___   8oz of water before lunch ___   8oz of water before dinner ___

This Morning's Self-Hypnosis | Round 1: Week 1—Fundamentals

Time you start: _____   Starting Stress Level (0–10): _____   Ending Stress Level (0–10): _____

This Afternoon's Self-Hypnosis | Round 2: Week 1—Fundamentals

Time you start: _____   Starting Stress Level (0–10): _____   Ending Stress Level (0–10): _____

This Evening's Self-Hypnosis | Round 3: Week 1—Fundamentals

Time you start: _____   Starting Stress Level (0–10): _____   Ending Stress Level (0–10): _____

Listen to this week's assigned hypnotherapy recording (found at www.CloseYourEyesLoseWeight.com): ☐

Tomorrow's Meal Planning

Breakfast	Snack	Lunch	Snack	Dinner

Check here when tomorrow's meals have been made or ordered: ☐

Visit www.CloseYourEyesLoseWeight.com and share your wins with our community: ☐

WEEK 1 LOG

TRACK YOUR PROGRESS

TODAY

Weight	Measurements	How Do You Feel in Your Clothes?	What's Your Energy Level?
	Neck: Waist:		
	Chest: Hips:	1 2 3 4 5	1 2 3 4 5
	(L) Arm (L) Thigh:		
	(R) Arm (R) Thigh:		

Write down any negative thoughts, immediately cross them
out, and replace them with a positive thought.

CANCEL-CANCEL BOX

[PRO TIP] Stay neutral. Get curious!

How Will You Conjure Up Additional Energy When Needed?

10 jumping jacks ___   Shout hypno-affirmations ___   Other ___

Water

8oz of water before breakfast ___   8oz of water before lunch ___   8oz of water before dinner ___

This Morning's Self-Hypnosis | Round 1: Week 1–Fundamentals

Time you start: _____   Starting Stress Level (0–10): _____   Ending Stress Level (0–10): _____

This Afternoon's Self-Hypnosis | Round 2: Week 1–Fundamentals

Time you start: _____   Starting Stress Level (0–10): _____   Ending Stress Level (0–10): _____

This Evening's Self-Hypnosis | Round 3: Week 1–Fundamentals

Time you start: _____   Starting Stress Level (0–10): _____   Ending Stress Level (0–10): _____

Listen to this week's assigned hypnotherapy recording (found at www.CloseYourEyesLoseWeight.com): ☐

Tomorrow's Meal Planning

Breakfast	Snack	Lunch	Snack	Dinner

Check here when tomorrow's meals have been made or ordered: ☐

Visit www.CloseYourEyesLoseWeight.com and share your wins with our community: ☐

WEEK 1 LOG

TRACK YOUR PROGRESS

TODAY

Weight	Measurements	How Do You Feel in Your Clothes?	What's Your Energy Level?
	Neck: Waist:		
	Chest: Hips:	1 2 3 4 5	1 2 3 4 5
	(L) Arm (L) Thigh:		
	(R) Arm (R) Thigh:		

Write down any negative thoughts, immediately cross them out, and replace them with a positive thought.

CANCEL-CANCEL BOX

[PRO TIP] Stay neutral. Get curious!

How Will You Conjure Up Additional Energy When Needed?

10 jumping jacks ___   Shout hypno-affirmations ___   Other ___

Water

8oz of water before breakfast ___   8oz of water before lunch ___   8oz of water before dinner ___

This Morning's Self-Hypnosis | Round 1: Week 1—Fundamentals

Time you start: _____   Starting Stress Level (0–10): _____   Ending Stress Level (0–10): _____

This Afternoon's Self-Hypnosis | Round 2: Week 1—Fundamentals

Time you start: _____   Starting Stress Level (0–10): _____   Ending Stress Level (0–10): _____

This Evening's Self-Hypnosis | Round 3: Week 1—Fundamentals

Time you start: _____   Starting Stress Level (0–10): _____   Ending Stress Level (0–10): _____

Listen to this week's assigned hypnotherapy recording (found at www.CloseYourEyesLoseWeight.com): ☐

Tomorrow's Meal Planning

Breakfast	Snack	Lunch	Snack	Dinner

Check here when tomorrow's meals have been made or ordered: ☐

Visit www.CloseYourEyesLoseWeight.com and share your wins with our community: ☐

WEEK 1 LOG

TRACK YOUR PROGRESS

TODAY

Weight	Measurements		How Do You Feel in Your Clothes?	What's Your Energy Level?
	Neck:	Waist:		
	Chest:	Hips:	1 2 3 4 5	1 2 3 4 5
	(L) Arm	(L) Thigh:		
	(R) Arm	(R) Thigh:		

Write down any negative thoughts, immediately cross them out, and replace them with a positive thought.

CANCEL-CANCEL BOX

[PRO TIP] Stay neutral. Get curious!

How Will You Conjure Up Additional Energy When Needed?

10 jumping jacks ___   Shout hypno-affirmations ___   Other ___

Water

8oz of water before breakfast ___   8oz of water before lunch ___   8oz of water before dinner ___

This Morning's Self-Hypnosis | Round 1: Week 1—Fundamentals

Time you start: _____   Starting Stress Level (0–10): _____   Ending Stress Level (0–10): _____

This Afternoon's Self-Hypnosis | Round 2: Week 1—Fundamentals

Time you start: _____   Starting Stress Level (0–10): _____   Ending Stress Level (0–10): _____

This Evening's Self-Hypnosis | Round 3: Week 1—Fundamentals

Time you start: _____   Starting Stress Level (0–10): _____   Ending Stress Level (0–10): _____

Listen to this week's assigned hypnotherapy recording (found at www.CloseYourEyesLoseWeight.com): ☐

Tomorrow's Meal Planning

Breakfast	Snack	Lunch	Snack	Dinner

Check here when tomorrow's meals have been made or ordered: ☐

Visit www.CloseYourEyesLoseWeight.com and share your wins with our community: ☐

CHAPTER 5

. . . .

Week 2–
Limiting Beliefs That
Have to Go

I t's time to discuss limiting *subconscious* beliefs about your ability to lose weight. If your **conscious** mind wants one thing (to lose weight) and your subconscious mind believes something else (it's unsafe to lose weight), your subconscious beliefs will beat out your conscious desires, every time.

It is important to unearth subconscious limiting beliefs because, whether you're aware of them or not, they're still at the helm of every decision you make (or do not make). If you're not aware of them, you cannot change them. Once you have this awareness, you can negotiate a new way of being. Once your conscious desires and your subconscious beliefs are in alignment, you will be free to live a life of design, rather than one by default!

The first step is to understand that your subconscious beliefs are shaping your reality. I always ask my clients why they believe their previous weight loss efforts failed. But I ask them twice . . . First, I ask their conscious mind before the hypnosis session starts. Then I ask them again once they are deep in hypnosis, when I know their subconscious will be answering. In this chart, you'll be able to compare the most common (from top to bottom) subconscious beliefs versus conscious beliefs about why losing weight has failed in the past.

Conscious beliefs for why weight loss failed in the past	Subconscious beliefs for why weight loss failed in the past
emotional eating	**"I'm not good enough"**: I'm a failure; I'm weak; I'm not worth taking care of; I'm not worthy of being thin and loving my body; I'm a loser.
eating when bored	**"It's in my genes"**: I'll always be overweight; I'm meant to be overweight because my whole family is obese; women in our family can't lose weight if we're over fifty.
carb addiction	**"It's not pleasurable to eat healthy"**: Junk food tastes better; healthy living is not fun; eating out is more enjoyable than cooking; fruits and vegetables are not as tasty; veggies are a punishment; nothing is tastier than carbs; good-tasting food is love.
sugar addiction	**"It's too *hard* to eat healthfully"**: Dieting takes so much planning and time; healthy foods are expensive and take too much time to prepare.
negative self-talk	**"I just can't do it"**: I can't change anything so there's no use in trying; I can't be healthy; I don't have faith in myself; I've started and stopped so many times; I'm not strong enough to stick to anything long enough to lose weight; even if I lose weight I'll never keep it off.

Conscious beliefs for why weight loss failed in the past	Subconscious beliefs for why weight loss failed in the past
meal planning/ cooking	"I don't want attention": It's not safe to have a physically attractive body; my weight is safe; the bigger I am, the less attention I get; my weight keeps me safe and hidden so no one will give me sexual attention.
binge eating	"I'm ugly" or "I'm unattractive."
hating my body	"I eat [insert processed food] to escape from [insert source of stress]."
friend/family sabotage	"I have no self-control."
stress	"I don't have time to exercise."
lack of sleep	"I don't deserve a body that I'm proud of."

Isn't the information in this chart fascinating? As you can see, the subconscious more often expresses deep pain such as "I don't have faith in myself," whereas the conscious mind often gives more surface reasonings like "carb addiction." There is also some crossover, of course. For example, emotional eating (the number one conscious mind answer) is clearly an *effect* of not feeling good enough (the number one subconscious mind answer). The subconscious mind knows the truth. For example, the real reason a client of mine struggled to lose weight in the past was because she had the *subconscious* belief that "women in my family can't lose weight when they're over fifty," not because of the second helpings (which her conscious mind believed was the culprit). The second helpings might be happening, but they are an effect, not a cause. Once my client realized this, she was able to do the work to heal the *actual* issue. Let's look at another cause-and-effect relationship.

Round 1

Cause = Feeling of not being good enough

Effect = Emotional eating

Next, the effect becomes the cause.

Round 2

Cause = Emotional eating

Effect = Weight gain, lethargy, a mindset of "I never stick to what I set out to do, I'm a failure."

Then the weight gain and feeling like a failure feed back into the feeling of not being good enough. This is a figure eight, which feeds into itself and loops back around.

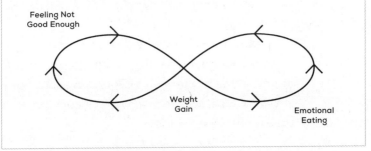

Feeling Not Good Enough

Weight Gain

Emotional Eating

Most people believe if they lose the weight, they'll stop feeling like a failure. The reality is that when you stop feeling like a failure (subconsciously), you'll finally be able to lose the weight.

This is why self-love isn't just a nice idea when coupled with weight loss initiatives; it's an absolute necessity. It can be tremendously helpful (although it isn't always necessary) to understand where your limiting beliefs around food, exercise, and weight loss **first began**. These are some of the more common sources I've heard from clients:

- Childhood trauma
- Family loss
- Family pressure
- Passed down in family, generation after generation
- Feeling different from and ostracized by one's peers
- Feeling overwhelmed with family and work commitments
- Failing at previous attempts to lose weight
- Financial challenges
- Unwanted attention
- Sexual abuse
- One's own insecurities
- "I'm not even sure where or when my limiting beliefs began."
  - If you also don't know where or when your limiting beliefs around food or weight began, once you listen to chapter five's hypnosis recording at www.CloseYourEyesLoseWeight.com, you'll have a much better idea.

Our Parents:
To Blame or Not to Blame?

Over the years I've noticed a tendency for limiting beliefs about food and our bodies to come from **Mom** more than anyone else in the family—which isn't surprising. Historically, the mother has always been the one who is cooking, food shopping, and making sure we're fed. She is therefore the one who was most likely to express love through food. No matter how our parents treated us, the subconscious wants to honor our parents often by choosing certain ways to be just like them, ways our conscious mind would never have agreed to if it had been given a vote. The subconscious believes that by "honoring" our parents through these traits it also increases our chances of being loved and therefore protected and cared for. It would feel subconsciously cruel to be thinner than Mom, or healthier than Mom, to be seen as looking down on her unhelpful recipes, or to not understand her plight of struggling with her weight all her life.

Of course, things could change for future generations now that more parents are sharing cooking and food shopping responsibilities, but for now the idea that "Mom is why I'm overweight" is certainly a common thread. Why is this important? Oftentimes, human beings want someone to blame for our own shortcomings, and I've noticed when clients first realize their subconscious challenges with weight loss stem back to Mom that their conscious minds have a desire to blame her for their current challenges with food and weight.

The fact of the matter, though, is Mom learned these beliefs, habits, and traits from someone else, too. And it's typically not a great use of time to sit around being angry with Grandma because *she* learned it from someone, too . . . And I know you don't have time to be mad at your great-great-nonna.

When we find out the "source" of our limiting or unhelpful beliefs, it is much more powerful to send them love for the struggles they faced. Forgive them and lovingly separate yourself from those anti-quated beliefs (this week's recording will show you how). While these challenges from the past might not be your *fault*, you are the only one who can change them now. When you take responsibility for cleaning up your subconscious, you pass on health-ier beliefs and habits to the next generation, who learn by observing your new and improved behav-iors. Take a nice, deep letting-go breath and recog-nize that you have the power to stop generational wounding. That is incredibly powerful.

And Dad, you're not getting let off the hook so easily. While many clients can trace "food is love" or "I love my mom too much to shame her by being skinnier than her" beliefs back to their moms, many clients can trace their first experi-ence of body shaming back to their dads. "If you can pinch an inch, it's time for a diet," said a dad to his twelve-year-old daughter as he squeezed the skin above his own hips, both to demonstrate how thin he was . . . and simultaneously point out how much more skin his daughter had. The result for the client? Body dysmorphia for the next fifteen years until she had her first hypnotherapy session. One comment resulted in more than a decade of need-less suffering. That might sound extreme, but it's a benign example compared to what many of my clients have experienced. And of course, it wasn't just one comment; it was the *first* of a lifetime of similar comments that made the first wound worse over time.

If you're a parent now (or wish to be in the future) and know you grew up surrounded by antiquated limiting beliefs and unhelpful actions, you're doing yourself and the next generation a massive favor by reading this book and taking responsibility for your subconscious mind. I'm so proud of you! Even though it's not your fault—and it's not even necessarily the fault of the person who taught it to you, either—you're going to help set the next generation of your family free. Often, we'll do for others what we won't do for ourselves, so another great way to beat Resistance when it shows up is to remind yourself, "I'm not just doing this for myself, I'm doing this for my kids." You'll be happily met with a surge of motivation to get back on track with upgrading and reconditioning your subconscious.

The last thing I'll say about parental influence is this: we won't get it right 100 percent of the time. As parents, we are going to occasionally slip up and say something unhelpful to our kids, something that was programmed into our brains when we were kids ourselves. Even if our kids grow up with some unhelpful beliefs and limiting thoughts, they'll still be the first generation to ever grow up with far *fewer* of them because we're the first humans in a long,

long time (perhaps ever)[42] to make cleaning up our subconscious minds a priority. If they continue to do the same as adults, they'll pass on even *less* subconscious junk to *their* kids. Think about the kind of human beings who will be walking this earth in two generations' time if we all commit to cleaning up our subconscious minds together, today.

As mentioned in chapter one, the subconscious always believes it's helping you. Even with the most wayward thinking and unhelpful habits imprinted in your subconscious blueprint, it still believes it is helping you. These beliefs cannot be transformed until the subconscious is satisfied that the ways in which it believes it is helping you will still be met. Here are some examples shared by Grace Spacers where their subconscious mind had a belief it felt was helping them but wasn't. In bold I've added examples of "reframes," which are ways of making the subconscious mind see this differently where you can get the result you want (buy-in from the subconscious to help you lose weight) and it still gets what it wants (to keep you safe). This will give you ideas on how you can reframe your own subconscious limiting beliefs while listening to this week's hypnosis audio recording:

- My subconscious belief thought it took less effort to hold on to my negative belief than to change it for a positive one. **Reframe: It's a lot more work to combat health issues in the future than it is to support**

---

42 In chapter three of *Close Your Eyes, Get Free* you can learn about how hypnosis was used in ancient Egyptian and druid cultures.

your health through optimal eating now. Choose being healthy now.

- My subconscious belief thought people would like me if I put their needs and feelings ahead of my own. **Reframe:** When you put yourself first, you have more energy to give to others. No one can drink from an empty cup. Fill up your cup first.

- My subconscious belief thought if I couldn't depend on the people in my life, I could at least depend on food to make me feel good. **Reframe:** You cannot change other people and resentment only hurts you. Release expectations of others and be the best you can be for yourself. Unhelpful foods are punishment; reward yourself with nourishing foods.

- My subconscious belief thought I could do everything on my own and handle anything. **Reframe:** You'll thrive for a lot longer by making helpful choices that are in your best interest now.

- My subconscious belief thought it protected me from failure and disappointment because being overweight became part of my personality. **Reframe:** The biggest disappointment of all is regret. You want to avoid the pain of regret at all costs. Go for your bold, beautiful life. Learn valuable lessons along the way, and you will avoid the pain of regret.

- My subconscious belief thought it protected me from all the unwanted attention. **Reframe:** If you hide because of an abuser's actions, they win. The courage to live an incredible life is within you. Find it now. You are worthy.

- My subconscious belief thought it protected me from punishment. **Reframe:** Unhelpful foods *are* a punishment. They steal our health and vitality. Reward yourself by claiming your rightful state of vibrant health.
- My subconscious belief thought it gave me an excuse, "Well, this is just how it is, and this is how I am." **Reframe:** Who decides "how you are"? Are you going to let others define you? If you want to be safe, you have to be in control. To be in control, you and you alone can define "how you are." Choose health. Choose happiness.
- My subconscious belief thought it kept me safe. **Reframe:** It is dangerous to be unhealthy. It is safe to eat helpful foods, to chew, to drink water, to stop eating when 90 percent satisfied, to move your body twenty minutes per day. These are your greatest insurance policies for a healthy, long life.
- My subconscious belief thought it kept me humble. **Reframe:** The thought "all God's children are magnificent because they were created by God" shows reverence for the body you were gifted. To eat unhelpful foods, to remain immobile, is to squander this divine gift. Show gratitude for your God-given body by treating your body kindly: eat helpful foods and move for twenty minutes per day.
- My subconscious belief thought it was giving me love. **Reframe:** Those old, unhelpful actions were a punishment. To show yourself love, stand in front of the mirror and say ten kind things to yourself, about yourself, right now. Feel your heart opening wide. You are worthy of love and respect just as you are.

If the subconscious believes it is keeping you safe and humble, and that it's protecting you from failure and disappointment, it's not going to give those things up lightly. The subconscious thinks it's doing important work by making sure the weight stays on. You have to prove to it that you are going to meet these needs of being safe and humble in other ways. During this week's hypnosis recording, there will be an opportunity for you to transform your limiting beliefs. After listening to it the first time, refer to the reframe list for ideas on how to reframe limiting beliefs so you'll have them handy for the second time you listen to the recording this week.

. . . .

Who Am I Without This Struggle?

Here is a very common limiting subconscious belief and how to reframe it:

"I've always been overweight. I've always had this struggle. I honestly don't know who I would be without it. I don't know what I would talk about or think about. I don't know how I would shop. I don't know what I would complain about. If I lose weight, I'll lose who I am. I'll lose my identity. I'll be lost."

If this belief exists in the subconscious mind, it's genuinely understandable. The subconscious (and Resistance) hate change. But (and bear with me, I'm going to get a little woo-woo here, but this topic calls for it) the truth is, you are more than the sum of your past problems. You are more than your body, even though it is miraculous and beautiful. You are more than your name, than your possessions, than your career, than your family life. At your core, you are infinite potential. You are boundless. You are perfection incarnate. You are consciousness.

The ego might be terrified of losing its overweight "identity" because it can't yet conceive of what it would be like to live in a body that weighs significantly less. Learning to dig deep into the truth of who you are *now* will allow you to love who you are when you reach your destination, as well as for every single step of the journey, and beyond it.

This week's hypnosis recording addresses this, and I so look forward to you leaning into the truth that you are so much more than your struggle. This is just something you're doing. You are a human *being*, not a human *doing*. **You** are the being-ness that is witnessing this weight loss. The you that is witnessing this transformation is unchangeable. Take a nice, deep letting-go breath and trust that you are worthy and deserving of witnessing these transformations in your body, mind, and spirit. Because you are infinite, the part of you experiencing weight loss is one tiny piece of who you are. In this week's hypnosis recording, you'll be able to reconcile subconscious fears about changing identity when you tap into the truth that your identity is beyond description. This means that however you choose to present yourself to the world is just a sliver of who you are, just a fragment of your essence. And if you choose to present that fragment of your essence in a more toned body,

> well, that is your prerogative, and it does nothing to change the magnificence of who you always have been and always will be.

Now that we have dissected popular limiting subconscious beliefs, it's time to discuss your everyday language. When it comes to weight loss, I've heard a lot of clients say, "I'm struggling with _____," or "It's so hard to _____." If you keep talking about what you're "struggling" with or what's "hard," you're programming yourself to struggle and for it to be hard! This isn't about negating feelings or solving everything with a blanket statement such as "Everything is easy if I just think it is." It's simply about choosing your language so you're focused on what you *do* want instead of what you don't want. Instead of saying, "I'm struggling with _____," use "I'm looking forward to improving _____."

When you become aware of the power of language and you start to listen to people around you, you realize 99 percent of people are constantly focused on what they don't want; it's what they spend all day talking about and thinking about. Even though they think they're talking about progress, they're talking about their problems, and in doing so are etching those problems deeper into their neural pathways.

Applying this to weight loss, you must focus on the body you desire to have. To get the body you want, you must love the body you have, yes, but you must also *visualize* the body you want. You must make it real, to hold the visual, to set a neurological framework, a precedent, so that your mind can get used to what it's like for you to be that new size. For most people, it is much easier to visualize the body they desire while in hypnosis.

Positive Versus Negative

I easily could have said, "For most people it's *harder* to visualize the body they want using their conscious mind." But I said instead, "It's much easier for most people to visualize the body they desire while in hypnosis." Both statements are true, though one focuses on the positive. You must speak the truth of what you want. Instead of saying, "I have so much weight left to lose," say, "I've already lost a few pounds and I'm so proud of myself. Every day I'm heading in the direction I want to go in, and it feels so good!"

A few phrases have got to go if you want to lose weight. You're no longer allowed to think them. You are definitely no longer allowed to say them, and if by force of habit they happen to pop up, you're going to say, "Cancel, cancel!" and replace them with what you want to be your reality.

For example, let's say you're putting on a top that used to fit perfectly. Now you're pulling it over your stomach and the thought that pops into your head is, **"I'm so fat."** That thought is not helping you lose weight. It is keeping the weight on. It is conditioning and programming you . . . It is hypnotizing you. Consider this: "The **first thought** that goes through your mind is what you have been **conditioned** to think. What **you think** next defines who **you are**."[43] If something like that comes into your mind accidentally, or out of habit, it's all good. All is not lost. You're working on creating new

---

43 Abby Luschei, "Your First Thought Does Not Define You," *Odyssey*, January 17, 2017, www.theodysseyonline.com/your-first-thought-does-define.

conditioning in your mind so there will be some overlap when old thoughts pop up before new thoughts take over. If those unhelpful thoughts show up, simply cancel them immediately so they don't strengthen those neural pathways. Say, for example, **"Cancel, cancel! Every day in every way I'm losing weight and feeling great."** You want to replace the negative language with a thought that is positive and believable so you can start to leave those old, useless, painful, harmful thoughts behind ASAP.

More examples of what has to go:

"Honey, do I look fat in this?" Not a question you're allowed to ask anymore. You know why? Because it has opened the possibility for a yes in your mind, regardless of what your partner says. That question is no longer allowed . . . even if your partner is wise enough not to take the bait.

"I'm so disgusting. Why do I bother?" Got to go. Start thinking positive thoughts: "Every day in every way I have more energy. Every day in every way I love myself more and more. I actually look really cute in this. My butt looks kinda nice in this!"

"I'm big boned." You might be, and if you are, great! Is affirming this with a negative connotation going to help you lose weight, feel great, and love your body? Nope. Replace it with "I love my strong body and enjoy getting healthier every day."

"Everyone in my family is obese." They might be. Is that thought, that conditioning, going to help you lose weight, feel great, and love yourself? Not a chance. Instead, say, "I'm honored to show my family what's possible. I'm worthy of being healthy. Every day in every way I'm losing weight and feeling great." I also suggest looking into the study of epigenetics, which teaches us that our genes are not our destiny.

The epigenome is the cellular material that sits on top of the genome (the complete set of genetic material present in a cell or organism). While epigenomes do not alter the genetic code, they direct genes to switch on (becoming active) or off (becoming dormant) through a variety of biological mechanisms. This intriguing finding means that your genetic heritage is not the primary determinant of your health, disease risk, or longevity . . . These changes in gene activity do not involve alterations to the genetic code, but are in great part determined by the choices we make . . . [D]iet, lifestyle, exercise, sleep habits, environmental factors, stress, and social relationships have all been shown to influence the expression of your genetic inheritance.[44]

Just because something *is*, doesn't necessarily mean you have to keep affirming it. You can affirm the positive things, the things that make you feel good, and the things that move you closer to your desired end goal.

Practice rewriting unhelpful thoughts. What are the last three negative thoughts you had about yourself, your weight, and your body? Write them down here, then "Cancel, cancel!" and flip the script!

1. a) Negative thought about yourself (write it and then cross it out):

   _____

   _____

   b) Say, "Cancel, cancel!"
   c) Positive thought to replace it with (use your

---

44 Donnie Yance, "Your Genes Are Not Your Destiny: The Science Of Epigenetics," DonnieYance.com, March 28, 2017, www.donnieyance.com/your-genes-are-not-your-destiny-the-science-of-epigenetics/.

emotions to *feel* the truth of this statement):

_____

_____

2. a) Negative thought about your weight (write it and then cross it out):

_____

_____

b) Say, "Cancel, cancel!"
c) Positive thought to replace it with (use your emotions to *feel* the truth of this statement):

_____

_____

3. a) Negative thought about your body (write it and then cross it out):

_____

_____

b) Say, "Cancel, cancel!"
c) Positive thought to replace it with (use your emotions to *feel* the truth of this statement):

_____

_____

This brings us to the final lesson of this chapter: **the subconscious will never let you become something you hate.**

Therefore, what shouldn't you hate? Or if hate is too strong a word to describe any lackluster sentiment, what can't you resent, dislike, look down upon, snub, feel jealousy or envy toward, be self-righteous toward, or criticize?

- Skinny people
- Healthy people
- Small-boned people

- People with good genes
- People who eat healthy food
- People who exercise
- People who appear to have it all together
- People who meal-prep religiously every Sunday night
- People who cook healthy meals for their kids
- Rich people . . . assuming you'd like to have some money

See where this is going?

Your subconscious is never going to allow you to have any of the things you want if you hate or resent or even moderately dislike the people who already have them.

Are you showing resentment or envy toward someone else who has something you want? Have you had thoughts like, "She won the gene lottery, good for her" (perhaps with a twinge of sarcasm), or "Must be nice to look like that" (perhaps with unveiled envy)?

Is this idea a radical shift for you? It's pretty much the opposite of what we're taught to do by society. We tend to scorn and scoff at or make fun of the people who have what we want so we can stop feeling bad about the fact that we don't have it. Unfortunately, that is the way to make sure we never get it. We're trained to make the "other" bad so we can feel better about ourselves. It is a protective mechanism.

Let's take Susan, for example. If Susan continues thinking negative thoughts about healthy, sexy, thin people, her subconscious will sabotage weight loss efforts all day long. Her subconscious is thinking, "If I become that, people will hate me. They'll think and say nasty things about me. They'll think I'm a bimbo. They'll think I got plastic surgery. How do I know people will think this about me? Because I've been thinking it about skinny people my whole life! It's safer to be big and appreciated for my humor and intellect." These thoughts aren't necessarily happening consciously, but they're certainly happening subconsciously. I've seen it time and time again with my clients. But the good news is, Susan doesn't have to choose! She can have it all—humor, intellect, health, and a body she loves.

If you want what someone else has, send them love. If you see someone with a gorgeous, toned body, rather than thinking, "Oh, I bet they have good genes. I bet they've had work done. I bet they have a personal trainer, must be nice," celebrate: "What a gorgeous, healthy body. I am so happy for that person, and I am loving my personal journey toward improving my health." Whatever it is that you desire to accomplish, start thinking positive thoughts toward the people who have already accomplished that and you'll get there faster—plus it feels good to support others! Send the healthy people around you even more healthiness! Send the woman with the beautiful bum even more beautiful bum-ness. Send the toned, strong folks love and appreciation for all they've done to cultivate such beautiful, healthy bods. You have to tell your subconscious what you want, and that it's safe for you to become that by showering love and appreciation on those souls who already have it.

Start showering love. Let's practice now:

Insert the name of someone fit, toned, and healthy, then repeat out loud ten times:

"_____, I'm proud of you, I thank you for being an example of what's possible, I send you love and even more of a sexy body and even more health and vitality!"

Now journal what you notice. How do you feel after those ten repetitions? How does this differ from how you used to feel when you thought about someone like that?

_____

_____

_____

You can use this with anyone who has a life you want—think of someone rich, or someone with a happy family, or someone who has a brilliant career. Send them love and support in their success.

Homework

A. Practice self-hypnosis three times a day, every day this week (right before breakfast, lunch, and dinner). Turn to page 20 for a reminder of how to do self-hypnosis or head to www. CloseYourEyesLoseWeight.com to follow along with a tutorial video.

Week 2 Hypno-affirmations—Limiting Beliefs

- I am worthy.
- I love how healthy food makes me feel.
- It is safe for me to lose weight and feel great.
- I am strong enough to do this.
- I deserve a body that I'm proud of.
- I am enough.

B. Listen to the "Week 2—Limiting Beliefs" hypnosis recording every day for the next week here: www. CloseYourEyesLoseWeight.com.

C. Use your journal pages daily to stay motivated, log your progress, and determine which pick-me-up hypno-affirmations you'll benefit from most.

You are now aware of your subconscious limiting beliefs and how they developed. Together, we've reframed those limiting beliefs into helpful, empowering beliefs. Your subconscious beliefs are now in alignment with your conscious desire to treat your body with love and respect. I'm so proud of you! It's time to go deeper. In chapter six, you're going to discover how to say yes to helpful foods and no to foods that don't support your body. Get ready to pass on the dessert without feeling deprived!

WEEK 2 LOG

TRACK YOUR PROGRESS

TODAY

Weight	Measurements	How Do You Feel in Your Clothes?	What's Your Energy Level?
	Neck: Waist:		
	Chest: Hips:	1 2 3 4 5	1 2 3 4 5
	(L) Arm (L) Thigh:		
	(R) Arm (R) Thigh:		

Write down any negative thoughts, immediately cross them out, and replace them with a positive thought.

CANCEL-CANCEL BOX

[PRO TIP] Stay neutral. Get curious!

How Will You Conjure Up Additional Energy When Needed?

10 jumping jacks ___   Shout hypno-affirmations ___   Other ___

Water

8oz of water before breakfast ___   8oz of water before lunch ___   8oz of water before dinner ___

This Morning's Self-Hypnosis | Round 1: Week 2—Limiting Beliefs

Time you start: _____   Starting Stress Level (0–10): _____   Ending Stress Level (0–10): _____

This Afternoon's Self-Hypnosis | Round 2: Week 2—Limiting Beliefs

Time you start: _____   Starting Stress Level (0–10): _____   Ending Stress Level (0–10): _____

This Evening's Self-Hypnosis | Round 3: Week 2—Limiting Beliefs

Time you start: _____   Starting Stress Level (0–10): _____   Ending Stress Level (0–10): _____

Listen to this week's assigned hypnotherapy recording (found at www.CloseYourEyesLoseWeight.com): ☐

Tomorrow's Meal Planning

Breakfast	Snack	Lunch	Snack	Dinner

Check here when tomorrow's meals have been made or ordered: ☐

Visit www.CloseYourEyesLoseWeight.com and share your wins with our community: ☐

WEEK 2 LOG

TRACK YOUR PROGRESS

TODAY

Weight	Measurements	How Do You Feel in Your Clothes?	What's Your Energy Level?
	Neck: Waist:		
	Chest: Hips:	1 2 3 4 5	1 2 3 4 5
	(L) Arm (L) Thigh:		
	(R) Arm (R) Thigh:		

Write down any negative thoughts, immediately cross them out, and replace them with a positive thought.

CANCEL-CANCEL BOX

. . . .

[PRO TIP] Stay neutral. Get curious!

. . . .

How Will You Conjure Up Additional Energy When Needed?

10 jumping jacks ___   Shout hypno-affirmations ___   Other ___

Water

8oz of water before breakfast ___   8oz of water before lunch ___   8oz of water before dinner ___

This Morning's Self-Hypnosis | Round 1: Week 2—Limiting Beliefs

Time you start: _____   Starting Stress Level (0–10): _____   Ending Stress Level (0–10): _____

This Afternoon's Self-Hypnosis | Round 2: Week 2—Limiting Beliefs

Time you start: _____   Starting Stress Level (0–10): _____   Ending Stress Level (0–10): _____

This Evening's Self-Hypnosis | Round 3: Week 2—Limiting Beliefs

Time you start: _____   Starting Stress Level (0–10): _____   Ending Stress Level (0–10): _____

Listen to this week's assigned hypnotherapy recording (found at www.CloseYourEyesLoseWeight.com): ☐

Tomorrow's Meal Planning

Breakfast	Snack	Lunch	Snack	Dinner

Check here when tomorrow's meals have been made or ordered: ☐

Visit www.CloseYourEyesLoseWeight.com and share your wins with our community: ☐

WEEK 2 LOG

TRACK YOUR PROGRESS

TODAY

Weight	Measurements	How Do You Feel in Your Clothes?	What's Your Energy Level?
	Neck: Waist:		
	Chest: Hips:	1 2 3 4 5	1 2 3 4 5
	(L) Arm (L) Thigh:		
	(R) Arm (R) Thigh:		

Write down any negative thoughts, immediately cross them out, and replace them with a positive thought.

CANCEL-CANCEL BOX

[PRO TIP] Stay neutral. Get curious!

How Will You Conjure Up Additional Energy When Needed?

10 jumping jacks ___   Shout hypno-affirmations ___   Other ___

Water

8oz of water before breakfast ___   8oz of water before lunch ___   8oz of water before dinner ___

This Morning's Self-Hypnosis | Round 1: Week 2–Limiting Beliefs

Time you start: _____   Starting Stress Level (0–10): _____   Ending Stress Level (0–10): _____

This Afternoon's Self-Hypnosis | Round 2: Week 2–Limiting Beliefs

Time you start: _____   Starting Stress Level (0–10): _____   Ending Stress Level (0–10): _____

This Evening's Self-Hypnosis | Round 3: Week 2–Limiting Beliefs

Time you start: _____   Starting Stress Level (0–10): _____   Ending Stress Level (0–10): _____

Listen to this week's assigned hypnotherapy recording (found at www.CloseYourEyesLoseWeight.com): ☐

Tomorrow's Meal Planning

Breakfast	Snack	Lunch	Snack	Dinner

Check here when tomorrow's meals have been made or ordered: ☐

Visit www.CloseYourEyesLoseWeight.com and share your wins with our community: ☐

WEEK 2 LOG

TRACK YOUR PROGRESS

TODAY

Weight	Measurements	How Do You Feel in Your Clothes?	What's Your Energy Level?
	Neck: Waist:		
	Chest: Hips:	1 2 3 4 5	1 2 3 4 5
	(L) Arm (L) Thigh:		
	(R) Arm (R) Thigh:		

Write down any negative thoughts, immediately cross them out, and replace them with a positive thought.

CANCEL-CANCEL BOX

[PRO TIP] Stay neutral. Get curious!

How Will You Conjure Up Additional Energy When Needed?

10 jumping jacks ___   Shout hypno-affirmations ___   Other ___

Water

8oz of water before breakfast ___   8oz of water before lunch ___   8oz of water before dinner ___

This Morning's Self-Hypnosis | Round 1: Week 2–Limiting Beliefs

Time you start: _____   Starting Stress Level (0–10): _____   Ending Stress Level (0–10): _____

This Afternoon's Self-Hypnosis | Round 2: Week 2–Limiting Beliefs

Time you start: _____   Starting Stress Level (0–10): _____   Ending Stress Level (0–10): _____

This Evening's Self-Hypnosis | Round 3: Week 2–Limiting Beliefs

Time you start: _____   Starting Stress Level (0–10): _____   Ending Stress Level (0–10): _____

Listen to this week's assigned hypnotherapy recording (found at www.CloseYourEyesLoseWeight.com): ☐

Tomorrow's Meal Planning

Breakfast	Snack	Lunch	Snack	Dinner

Check here when tomorrow's meals have been made or ordered: ☐

Visit www.CloseYourEyesLoseWeight.com and share your wins with our community: ☐

WEEK 2 LOG

TRACK YOUR PROGRESS

TODAY

Weight	Measurements	How Do You Feel in Your Clothes?	What's Your Energy Level?
	Neck: Waist:		
	Chest: Hips:	1 2 3 4 5	1 2 3 4 5
	(L) Arm (L) Thigh:		
	(R) Arm (R) Thigh:		

Write down any negative thoughts, immediately cross them out, and replace them with a positive thought.

CANCEL-CANCEL BOX

· ·

[PRO TIP] Stay neutral. Get curious!

· ·

How Will You Conjure Up Additional Energy When Needed?

10 jumping jacks __   Shout hypno-affirmations __   Other __

Water

8oz of water before breakfast __   8oz of water before lunch __   8oz of water before dinner __

This Morning's Self-Hypnosis | Round 1: Week 2—Limiting Beliefs

Time you start: _____   Starting Stress Level (0–10): _____   Ending Stress Level (0–10): _____

This Afternoon's Self-Hypnosis | Round 2: Week 2—Limiting Beliefs

Time you start: _____   Starting Stress Level (0–10): _____   Ending Stress Level (0–10): _____

This Evening's Self-Hypnosis | Round 3: Week 2—Limiting Beliefs

Time you start: _____   Starting Stress Level (0–10): _____   Ending Stress Level (0–10): _____

Listen to this week's assigned hypnotherapy recording (found at www.CloseYourEyesLoseWeight.com): ☐

Tomorrow's Meal Planning

Breakfast	Snack	Lunch	Snack	Dinner

Check here when tomorrow's meals have been made or ordered: ☐

Visit www.CloseYourEyesLoseWeight.com and share your wins with our community: ☐

WEEK 2 LOG

DATE: __ / __ / __

TRACK YOUR PROGRESS

TODAY

Weight	Measurements	How Do You Feel in Your Clothes?	What's Your Energy Level?
	Neck: Waist:		
	Chest: Hips:	1 2 3 4 5	1 2 3 4 5
	(L) Arm (L) Thigh:		
	(R) Arm (R) Thigh:		

Write down any negative thoughts, immediately cross them out, and replace them with a positive thought.

CANCEL-CANCEL BOX

[PRO TIP] Stay neutral. Get curious!

How Will You Conjure Up Additional Energy When Needed?

10 jumping jacks __   Shout hypno-affirmations __   Other __

Water

8oz of water before breakfast __   8oz of water before lunch __   8oz of water before dinner __

This Morning's Self-Hypnosis | Round 1: Week 2–Limiting Beliefs

Time you start: _____   Starting Stress Level (0–10): _____   Ending Stress Level (0–10): _____

This Afternoon's Self-Hypnosis | Round 2: Week 2–Limiting Beliefs

Time you start: _____   Starting Stress Level (0–10): _____   Ending Stress Level (0–10): _____

This Evening's Self-Hypnosis | Round 3: Week 2–Limiting Beliefs

Time you start: _____   Starting Stress Level (0–10): _____   Ending Stress Level (0–10): _____

Listen to this week's assigned hypnotherapy recording (found at www.CloseYourEyesLoseWeight.com): ☐

Tomorrow's Meal Planning

Breakfast	Snack	Lunch	Snack	Dinner

Check here when tomorrow's meals have been made or ordered: ☐

Visit www.CloseYourEyesLoseWeight.com and share your wins with our community: ☐

WEEK 2 LOG

TRACK YOUR PROGRESS

TODAY

Weight	Measurements	How Do You Feel in Your Clothes?	What's Your Energy Level?
	Neck: Waist:		
	Chest: Hips:	1 2 3 4 5	1 2 3 4 5
	(L) Arm (L) Thigh:		
	(R) Arm (R) Thigh:		

Write down any negative thoughts, immediately cross them out, and replace them with a positive thought.

CANCEL-CANCEL BOX

[PRO TIP] Stay neutral. Get curious!

How Will You Conjure Up Additional Energy When Needed?

10 jumping jacks ___   Shout hypno-affirmations ___   Other ___

Water

8oz of water before breakfast ___   8oz of water before lunch ___   8oz of water before dinner ___

This Morning's Self-Hypnosis | Round 1: Week 2–Limiting Beliefs

Time you start: _____   Starting Stress Level (0–10): _____   Ending Stress Level (0–10): _____

This Afternoon's Self-Hypnosis | Round 2: Week 2–Limiting Beliefs

Time you start: _____   Starting Stress Level (0–10): _____   Ending Stress Level (0–10): _____

This Evening's Self-Hypnosis | Round 3: Week 2–Limiting Beliefs

Time you start: _____   Starting Stress Level (0–10): _____   Ending Stress Level (0–10): _____

Listen to this week's assigned hypnotherapy recording (found at www.CloseYourEyesLoseWeight.com): ☐

Tomorrow's Meal Planning

Breakfast	Snack	Lunch	Snack	Dinner

Check here when tomorrow's meals have been made or ordered: ☐

Visit www.CloseYourEyesLoseWeight.com and share your wins with our community: ☐

CHAPTER 6

· · · · · · · · · · · · · · · · · ·

Week 3–
Intuitive Eating

Our opinions are based on our subconscious programming and our current circumstances. If our subconscious minds change, our opinions change. For example, before hypnosis, someone with a sugar addiction might believe: "Sugar is everything, I want dessert with every meal. I deserve to eat things that taste indulgent and amazing." After hypnosis, the same person might think: "Sugar actually isn't delicious. It's kind of disgusting. It's way too sweet, and consuming it makes me feel terrible. I don't want it. Get it away from me!" Two different opinions held by the same person, just weeks apart.

Adding another layer, take a moment to consider how opinions can be backed by facts and *still* be opinions. How can that be? Facts are facts!

Well, there are facts to back up why it's good to put bacon on everything.

There are facts that say bacon causes heart disease.

There are facts that say some red wine is good.

There are facts that say alcohol kills brain cells.

There are facts that say fat in food causes fat in bodies.

There are facts that say fat is required for healthy brain functionality.

There are facts that say sugar is bad for us, so use sweeteners.

There are facts that say artificial sweeteners cause innumerable diseases.

There are facts that say vegetables will solve all your health problems.

There are facts that say nightshade vegetables must be avoided by people with autoimmune disease.

And what do we do with all this contradictory yet proven information? We all pick our favorite facts that fit in with our current worldview and then we defend them mercilessly. There might even be genuine, irrefutable science that proves one way of eating is healthier or is better for the environment, but if the findings of that science in any way go against our personal belief systems or, honestly, convenience, well, the truth is rarely enough to change human behavior. We typically become set in our ways and then defend those ways as the only "right" way. Which facts we make our favorites (i.e., the ones we choose to believe over others) are largely informed by the people we hang out with, where we live, what we care about, and honestly what we want to do.

What you genuinely believe is healthy or good to eat is likely deeply offensive to someone, somewhere in the world. Plus, with food allergies and sensitivities on the rise, what's healthy for one person, regardless of that person's opinions or beliefs, is different from what's healthy for someone else. When you combine the confusion of everyone choosing their "favorite facts" according to preconceived worldviews, thousands of different diet books, and individual food sensitivities, how the heck do we know what to eat? The answer is, you combine blood tests and intuitive eating.

Blood Tests

Blood tests will tell you what you are allergic to and sensitive to so you can stop eating them regardless of your opinions and your taste buds' preferences. While certainly an investment, if you can afford to get this done at least once to start with, you will be amazed at how much better you feel when you know what foods to omit from your diet. Why? Because if you eat food you are allergic to, you will have an allergic reaction. That is bad. Objectively bad. Not favorite facts bad. Continual allergic reactions over time can lead to chronic inflammation.[45] (You'll learn more about "leaky gut," which may be the reason for these allergies and sensitivities in a bit.)

You might think you have no food allergies—my forty-two-year-old client Jake didn't think he had any, and he had nine. NINE! But to him an "allergic reaction" is what happened to his neighbor when he was a kid; Evan was stung by a bee and rushed to the hospital in anaphylactic shock. Since nothing like this had ever happened to Jake, he assumed he didn't have any allergies. When Jake found out allergic reactions might look like bloating, extreme fatigue, dizziness, light-headedness, weight gain, rashes, he realized he had been expressing some version of these symptoms every day, for years. Once he received his blood test back and eliminated these nine foods from his diet, he not only lost weight much faster but also felt more energized and clearheaded than he had since he was a teenager.

If you've ever wondered if hidden allergies or sensitivities may be at the root of your weight gain or health issues, you might benefit from being on the lookout for a condition called "leaky gut." According to Healthline,

---

45 Lisa Esposito, "When You're Allergic to Almost Every Food," *U.S. News*, March 9, 2016, https://health.usnews.com/health-news/patient-advice/articles /2016-03-09/when-youre-allergic-to-almost-every-food.

Leaky gut, also known as increased intestinal permeability, is a digestive condition in which bacteria and toxins are able to "leak" through the intestinal wall. Mainstream medical professionals do not recognize leaky gut as a real condition. However, there is quite a bit of scientific evidence that leaky gut does exist and may be associated with multiple health problems.[46]

Jake's integrative physician explained to him that with leaky gut you can become sensitive or allergic to foods you eat often because food proteins are crossing the intestinal barrier and the body attacks the foreign agent with an immune response. That is the definition of a food allergy.

So Jake can eat gluten, cheese, and sugar without having an allergic response, but it doesn't make those foods "healthy," and they're **not helpful** to any weight loss goals. But at the present moment if he were to eat broccoli, onions, green beans, almonds, or ginger, he would be doubled over in pain because he has developed food sensitivities toward these foods over the years—which doesn't make these foods "unhealthy" for anyone else who doesn't have those same food sensitivities.

This is why intuitive eating, which we'll dive into in a moment, is so important. Just because Jake's body can't process celery or ginger or broccoli right now doesn't make them "bad foods."

If you have a history of disordered eating, referring to certain foods as "bad" food, "junk" food, "garbage," or "poison" might be triggering. Even for those

46 Becky Bell, "Is Leaky Gut Syndrome a Real Condition? An Unbiased Look," Healthline, February 2, 2017, www.healthline.com/nutrition/is-leaky-gut-real.

without a history of disordered eating, those terms might feel extreme to you. For others, these terms will be helpful in programming the subconscious to choose a different way of eating, and it won't be triggering at all. As always, please continue to view this book and all resources as a "choose your own adventure" by only choosing hypno-affirmations that will imprint your subconscious mind with the terms that are most helpful for *you*. More on this and aversion therapy on page 185.

The good news? Once you have data about any potential food allergies and sensitivities, you can use hypnotherapy to rewire your brain so you no longer crave or miss the foods that are **objectively** bad for you. You can also use hypnotherapy to overcome a fear of needles so blood work becomes a breeze!

Intuitive Eating

Intuitive eating is eating or not eating what's right for *you*, right now, in this moment. What's right for you in the morning might not be right for you in the afternoon. What your best friend is ordering for brunch might not be right for you, no matter how Instagrammable it looks. What's right for you in July might not be right for you in December. What's right for you might not look anything like what your past opinions and favorite facts would agree with. It doesn't matter. Your past opinions and favorite facts were formed before you committed to changing your life and to doing what it takes to get the results you're looking for.

If your past opinion was that cooking with lard is delicious (because your grandmother taught you how to cook, and that was her opinion—so watch it, Grace, you better not say one bad word about my granny!) but your intuition tells you lard is making you feel awful, you *have* to go with your intuition. Not what your mind tells you to eat, not what I tell you to eat, not what beloved Granny told you to eat—what your own *intuition* tells you. If you want the results you wrote down on your Intake Form, and I know you do, committing to eating intuitively will get you there. Letting go of past opinions and the "favorite facts" will get you there.

Here's a great explanation from Healthline of how you can use the subconscious mind to decide what's right for you:

> Intuitive eating is a philosophy of eating that makes you the expert of your body and its hunger signals . . . Essentially, it's the opposite of a traditional diet . . . It doesn't impose guidelines about what to avoid and what or when to eat . . . Instead, it teaches that you are the best person—the only person—to make those choices . . . To eat intuitively, you may need to relearn how to trust your body . . .To do that, you need to distinguish between physical and emotional hunger:
>
> - **Physical hunger.** This biological urge tells you to replenish nutrients. It builds gradually and has different signals, such as a growling stomach, fatigue, or irritability. It's satisfied when you eat any food.
> - **Emotional hunger.** This is driven by emotional need. Sadness, loneliness, and boredom are some of the feelings that can create cravings for

food, often comfort foods. Eating then causes
guilt and self-hatred.[47]

When I teach my clients intuitive eating at the subconscious level, it all becomes crystal clear. They understand what foods are making them feel sluggish, unhealthy, unhappy, disgusting, gross. They understand which foods their body is craving more of. They are able to tap into the power of intuitive eating when prepping their meals, when food shopping, when ordering at a restaurant. And most importantly, they are able to determine if they are experiencing a genuine sensation of hunger, or if an uncomfortable emotion is activated and it's attempting to soothe itself through the neurochemicals released by certain foods. In this week's hypnosis recording, you will learn how to train your brain to release any old, unhelpful opinions and learn to eat intuitively in a way that's right for you and your unique makeup.

Homework

A. Practice self-hypnosis three times a day, every day this week (right before breakfast, lunch, and dinner). Turn to page 20 for a reminder of how to do self-hypnosis or head to www.CloseYourEyesLoseWeight.com to follow along with a tutorial video.

---

47 Kerri-Ann Jennings, "A Quick Guide to Intuitive Eating," Healthline, June 25, 2019, www.healthline.com/nutrition/quick-guide-intuitive-eating#basics.

Week 3 Hypno-affirmations—Intuitive Eating

- Blood tests help me know which foods are best for me.
- My intuition knows which foods nourish me most.
- I take a deep breath and tune in before ordering food.
- I take a deep breath and tune in before buying food.
- I choose foods that support my long-term health.
- My body is a machine. Food is fuel. I only put the highest quality fuel into my machine.

B. Listen to the "Week 3—Intuitive Eating" hypnosis recording every day for the next week here: www. CloseYourEyesLoseWeight.com.

C. Use your journal pages daily to stay motivated, log your progress, and determine which pick-me-up hypno-affirmations you'll benefit from most.

. . . .

You've now learned how to replace opinions about food with the objective truth about what *your* body—and yours alone—needs. All thanks to blood tests and intuitive eating, which tell the story of what works for you and what doesn't. I'm sure you're feeling infinitely better already! As we go into week four, you'll learn how to do what many people consider impossible—crave exercise. Yes, it's not only possible, it is the expected outcome when you retrain your brain. I'll show you how.

TRACK YOUR PROGRESS

TODAY

Weight	Measurements	How Do You Feel in Your Clothes?	What's Your Energy Level?
	Neck: Waist:		
	Chest: Hips:	1 2 3 4 5	1 2 3 4 5
	(L) Arm (L) Thigh:		
	(R) Arm (R) Thigh:		

Write down any negative thoughts, immediately cross them out, and replace them with a positive thought.

CANCEL-CANCEL BOX

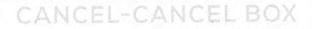

[PRO TIP] Stay neutral. Get curious!

How Will You Conjure Up Additional Energy When Needed?

10 jumping jacks ___   Shout hypno-affirmations ___   Other ___

Water

8oz of water before breakfast ___   8oz of water before lunch ___   8oz of water before dinner ___

This Morning's Self-Hypnosis | Round 1: Week 3—Intuitive Eating

Time you start: _____   Starting Stress Level (0–10): _____   Ending Stress Level (0–10): _____

This Afternoon's Self-Hypnosis | Round 2: Week 3—Intuitive Eating

Time you start: _____   Starting Stress Level (0–10): _____   Ending Stress Level (0–10): _____

This Evening's Self-Hypnosis | Round 3: Week 3—Intuitive Eating

Time you start: _____   Starting Stress Level (0–10): _____   Ending Stress Level (0–10): _____

Listen to this week's assigned hypnotherapy recording (found at www.CloseYourEyesLoseWeight.com): ☐

Tomorrow's Meal Planning

Breakfast	Snack	Lunch	Snack	Dinner

Check here when tomorrow's meals have been made or ordered: ☐

Visit www.CloseYourEyesLoseWeight.com and share your wins with our community: ☐

WEEK 3 LOG

TRACK YOUR PROGRESS

TODAY

Weight	Measurements	How Do You Feel in Your Clothes?	What's Your Energy Level?
	Neck: Waist:		
	Chest: Hips:	1 2 3 4 5	1 2 3 4 5
	(L) Arm (L) Thigh:		
	(R) Arm (R) Thigh:		

Write down any negative thoughts, immediately cross them out, and replace them with a positive thought.

CANCEL-CANCEL BOX

[PRO TIP] Stay neutral. Get curious!

How Will You Conjure Up Additional Energy When Needed?

10 jumping jacks ___   Shout hypno-affirmations ___   Other ___

Water

8oz of water before breakfast ___   8oz of water before lunch ___   8oz of water before dinner ___

This Morning's Self-Hypnosis | Round 1: Week 3–Intuitive Eating

Time you start: _____   Starting Stress Level (0–10): _____   Ending Stress Level (0–10): _____

This Afternoon's Self-Hypnosis | Round 2: Week 3–Intuitive Eating

Time you start: _____   Starting Stress Level (0–10): _____   Ending Stress Level (0–10): _____

This Evening's Self-Hypnosis | Round 3: Week 3–Intuitive Eating

Time you start: _____   Starting Stress Level (0–10): _____   Ending Stress Level (0–10): _____

Listen to this week's assigned hypnotherapy recording (found at www.CloseYourEyesLoseWeight.com): ☐

Tomorrow's Meal Planning

Breakfast	Snack	Lunch	Snack	Dinner

Check here when tomorrow's meals have been made or ordered: ☐

Visit www.CloseYourEyesLoseWeight.com and share your wins with our community: ☐

TRACK YOUR PROGRESS

TODAY

Weight	Measurements	How Do You Feel in Your Clothes?	What's Your Energy Level?
	Neck: Waist:		
	Chest: Hips:		
	(L) Arm (L) Thigh:	1 2 3 4 5	1 2 3 4 5
	(R) Arm (R) Thigh:		

Write down any negative thoughts, immediately cross them out, and replace them with a positive thought.

CANCEL-CANCEL BOX

[PRO TIP] Stay neutral. Get curious!

How Will You Conjure Up Additional Energy When Needed?

10 jumping jacks ___   Shout hypno-affirmations ___   Other ___

Water

8oz of water before breakfast ___   8oz of water before lunch ___   8oz of water before dinner ___

This Morning's Self-Hypnosis | Round 1: Week 3—Intuitive Eating

Time you start: _____   Starting Stress Level (0–10): _____   Ending Stress Level (0–10): _____

This Afternoon's Self-Hypnosis | Round 2: Week 3—Intuitive Eating

Time you start: _____   Starting Stress Level (0–10): _____   Ending Stress Level (0–10): _____

This Evening's Self-Hypnosis | Round 3: Week 3—Intuitive Eating

Time you start: _____   Starting Stress Level (0–10): _____   Ending Stress Level (0–10): _____

Listen to this week's assigned hypnotherapy recording (found at www.CloseYourEyesLoseWeight.com): ☐

Tomorrow's Meal Planning

Breakfast	Snack	Lunch	Snack	Dinner

Check here when tomorrow's meals have been made or ordered: ☐

Visit www.CloseYourEyesLoseWeight.com and share your wins with our community: ☐

WEEK 3 LOG

TRACK YOUR PROGRESS

TODAY

Weight	Measurements		How Do You Feel in Your Clothes?	What's Your Energy Level?
	Neck:	Waist:		
	Chest:	Hips:		
	(L) Arm	(L) Thigh:	1 2 3 4 5	1 2 3 4 5
	(R) Arm	(R) Thigh:		

Write down any negative thoughts, immediately cross them out, and replace them with a positive thought.

CANCEL-CANCEL BOX

[PRO TIP] Stay neutral. Get curious!

How Will You Conjure Up Additional Energy When Needed?

10 jumping jacks ___   Shout hypno-affirmations ___   Other ___

Water

8oz of water before breakfast ___   8oz of water before lunch ___   8oz of water before dinner ___

This Morning's Self-Hypnosis | Round 1: Week 3—Intuitive Eating

Time you start: _____   Starting Stress Level (0–10): _____   Ending Stress Level (0–10): _____

This Afternoon's Self-Hypnosis | Round 2: Week 3—Intuitive Eating

Time you start: _____   Starting Stress Level (0–10): _____   Ending Stress Level (0–10): _____

This Evening's Self-Hypnosis | Round 3: Week 3—Intuitive Eating

Time you start: _____   Starting Stress Level (0–10): _____   Ending Stress Level (0–10): _____

Listen to this week's assigned hypnotherapy recording (found at www.CloseYourEyesLoseWeight.com): ☐

Tomorrow's Meal Planning

Breakfast	Snack	Lunch	Snack	Dinner

Check here when tomorrow's meals have been made or ordered: ☐

Visit www.CloseYourEyesLoseWeight.com and share your wins with our community: ☐

WEEK 3 LOG

TRACK YOUR PROGRESS

TODAY

Weight	Measurements	How Do You Feel in Your Clothes?	What's Your Energy Level?
	Neck: Waist:		
	Chest: Hips:	1 2 3 4 5	1 2 3 4 5
	(L) Arm (L) Thigh:		
	(R) Arm (R) Thigh:		

Write down any negative thoughts, immediately cross them out, and replace them with a positive thought.

CANCEL-CANCEL BOX

[PRO TIP] Stay neutral. Get curious!

How Will You Conjure Up Additional Energy When Needed?

10 jumping jacks ___   Shout hypno-affirmations ___   Other ___

Water

8oz of water before breakfast ___   8oz of water before lunch ___   8oz of water before dinner ___

This Morning's Self-Hypnosis | Round 1: Week 3—Intuitive Eating

Time you start: _____   Starting Stress Level (0–10): _____   Ending Stress Level (0–10): _____

This Afternoon's Self-Hypnosis | Round 2: Week 3—Intuitive Eating

Time you start: _____   Starting Stress Level (0–10): _____   Ending Stress Level (0–10): _____

This Evening's Self-Hypnosis | Round 3: Week 3—Intuitive Eating

Time you start: _____   Starting Stress Level (0–10): _____   Ending Stress Level (0–10): _____

Listen to this week's assigned hypnotherapy recording (found at www.CloseYourEyesLoseWeight.com): ☐

Tomorrow's Meal Planning

Breakfast	Snack	Lunch	Snack	Dinner

Check here when tomorrow's meals have been made or ordered: ☐

Visit www.CloseYourEyesLoseWeight.com and share your wins with our community: ☐

WEEK 3 LOG

TRACK YOUR PROGRESS

TODAY

Weight	Measurements	How Do You Feel in Your Clothes?	What's Your Energy Level?
	Neck: Waist:		
	Chest: Hips:	1 2 3 4 5	1 2 3 4 5
	(L) Arm (L) Thigh:		
	(R) Arm (R) Thigh:		

Write down any negative thoughts, immediately cross them out, and replace them with a positive thought.

CANCEL-CANCEL BOX

. . . .

[PRO TIP] Stay neutral. Get curious!

. . . .

How Will You Conjure Up Additional Energy When Needed?

10 jumping jacks __   Shout hypno-affirmations __   Other __

Water

8oz of water before breakfast __   8oz of water before lunch __   8oz of water before dinner __

This Morning's Self-Hypnosis | Round 1: Week 3—Intuitive Eating

Time you start: _____   Starting Stress Level (0–10): _____   Ending Stress Level (0–10): _____

This Afternoon's Self-Hypnosis | Round 2: Week 3—Intuitive Eating

Time you start: _____   Starting Stress Level (0–10): _____   Ending Stress Level (0–10): _____

This Evening's Self-Hypnosis | Round 3: Week 3—Intuitive Eating

Time you start: _____   Starting Stress Level (0–10): _____   Ending Stress Level (0–10): _____

Listen to this week's assigned hypnotherapy recording (found at www.CloseYourEyesLoseWeight.com): ☐

Tomorrow's Meal Planning

Breakfast	Snack	Lunch	Snack	Dinner

Check here when tomorrow's meals have been made or ordered: ☐

Visit www.CloseYourEyesLoseWeight.com and share your wins with our community: ☐

TRACK YOUR PROGRESS

TODAY

Weight	Measurements	How Do You Feel in Your Clothes?	What's Your Energy Level?
	Neck: Waist:		
	Chest: Hips:		
	(L) Arm (L) Thigh:	1 2 3 4 5	1 2 3 4 5
	(R) Arm (R) Thigh:		

Write down any negative thoughts, immediately cross them out, and replace them with a positive thought.

CANCEL-CANCEL BOX

[PRO TIP] Stay neutral. Get curious!

How Will You Conjure Up Additional Energy When Needed?

10 jumping jacks ___   Shout hypno-affirmations ___   Other ___

Water

8oz of water before breakfast ___   8oz of water before lunch ___   8oz of water before dinner ___

This Morning's Self-Hypnosis | Round 1: Week 3—Intuitive Eating

Time you start: _____   Starting Stress Level (0–10): _____   Ending Stress Level (0–10): _____

This Afternoon's Self-Hypnosis | Round 2: Week 3—Intuitive Eating

Time you start: _____   Starting Stress Level (0–10): _____   Ending Stress Level (0–10): _____

This Evening's Self-Hypnosis | Round 3: Week 3—Intuitive Eating

Time you start: _____   Starting Stress Level (0–10): _____   Ending Stress Level (0–10): _____

Listen to this week's assigned hypnotherapy recording (found at www.CloseYourEyesLoseWeight.com): ☐

Tomorrow's Meal Planning

Breakfast	Snack	Lunch	Snack	Dinner

Check here when tomorrow's meals have been made or ordered: ☐

Visit www.CloseYourEyesLoseWeight.com and share your wins with our community: ☐

CHAPTER 7

· · · · · · · · · · · · · · ·

Week 4–
Training Your Brain to
Crave Exercise

"I had so much resistance to moving my body. Until I had a hypnotherapy session, I just thought I didn't exercise because I was 'lazy.' During my session, I realized that because my dad deserted our family when I was three years old and because he had been a bodybuilder, my subconscious was rebelling against exercise as a way to 'side with' my mom. I don't even have any conscious memories of my dad, yet I spent years hurting myself by being immobile because of this belief! Through the hypnosis session, I was able to let go of that. I spent a number of additional hypnotherapy sessions healing the feelings of abandonment and anger that were

> previously buried, and I now run a 5k every morning.
> I've decided to 'side with my mom' by being healthy
> so she has one less thing to worry about." —Alex M.,
> Quebec, Canada

We've arrived at the exercise chapter . . . and the groans are audible to me now from across time and space. ;) But take a nice, deep letting-go breath and put a smile on your face, this is going to be great! Again, I am not a personal trainer, so I'm not going to ask you to get out your yoga mat and do a hundred crunches right now, although you may choose to make that part of your daily routine after you master what this chapter's hypnosis will teach you.

Amelia, a Grace Spacer, asked, "I have a question about exercise. I enjoy it and it feels so good when I do it, but it's so hard to get myself to do any movement. How do I even get started? And then continue?"

Danette May is a world-renowned speaker and healthy-lifestyle expert who has helped millions of people through her principles of healing food, movement, and mindset. This is her response to Amelia:

> The key to movement is to drop into something you love.
> Whether it's running or dance or yoga, if it calls to you
> and you feel great when you do it, you're more likely to
> stick with it. Once you decide the type of movement that
> most fires you up, seek out a community of others who
> like the same things or who are going through the same
> healthy movement mindset shifts you are. There is power
> in support systems. When you have a tribe of people
> experiencing similar growth, you become both inspired

and unstoppable. Soon you'll find yourself trying new things and embracing that exercise is a reward for your body, not a punishment. Take that first step—you got this!

With Danette's wisdom in mind, this week you're going to discover the kind of movement your body most enjoys and then train your subconscious mind to do that for twenty minutes per day.

Here's the thing: Do you ever notice how people who exercise daily love it? I mean LOVE it. They're obsessed! They feel like something is wrong if they *don't* exercise. And the inverse is also true . . . that most people who don't exercise **hate** it. They avoid it like the plague.

In my experience, few people who have a neutral feeling toward exercise do it with any consistency.

The reason exercising feels so good for those who stick with it is because endorphins are released. According to WebMD, "Endorphins interact with the receptors in your brain that reduce your perception of pain. Endorphins also trigger a positive feeling in the body, similar to that of morphine."[48] The "runner's high" is a real high! Committed runners go out for a glorious five-mile run, come rain, sun, sleet, or snow, smiling from ear to ear while rocking out to music they love, because their body is so looking forward to the massive reward of that natural high.

These beautiful creatures (I'm not being sarcastic! Remember, we have to LOVE those who exercise so our subconscious will let us become one of them) might seem like mythical fairies to you now—with their high ponytails and green juices and vegan protein power bars tucked inside their leggings for a mid-run snack—but they're not. They're simply humans who've unlocked the natural

---

48 "Exercise and Depression," WebMD, accessed November 4, 2019, www. webmd.com/depression/guide/exercise-depression.

power of endorphins through exercise. And they've exercised enough times in a row that it became *habitual*, so much so that the release of endorphins through movement (not food) is *craved*.

Human beings have a built-in feel-good release of hormones whenever we do things that help our species to survive. We also have built-in major fear responses for anything perceived to be even a remote threat toward our survival. For the past chapters, you've been overcoming many of those innate fear responses that we no longer need in the modern world. Now, you're going to unlock the power of the endorphins that are naturally released with regular exercise so you can crave moving your body in a way that will help you to survive, thrive, and enjoy life for much longer.

> Remember, exercise releases feel-good neuro-chemicals because, in order for our species to continue to flourish, we have to exercise!

Many of my clients who exercise daily use this time to do their manifesting. It's how they access joy now. They look forward to it; it's their happiest time of the day. So here's the thing about training your subconscious brain to exercise: you have to go all in.

All in.

I'm not saying you have to go out and run a marathon tomorrow (in fact, you should not do that . . . more on this in a sec) but it's vital to exercise until it **feels good**. Once you get that release of endorphins, it becomes straightforward to tell the subconscious that you want more of it and to build a neural framework of experience that includes you moving your body on a daily basis.

According to Exercise.com, "The time it takes for endorphins to flood the body while exercising will vary from person to person.

For some people, as little as ten minutes of intense exercise will do the trick. For others, it takes as long as thirty minutes or more. Whatever the case may be, endorphins are one of those things that when they get released, you know."[49]

Some people need ten minutes, some need thirty, so this week (and every week morning forward) you're going to split the difference and train your subconscious mind to love and crave twenty minutes of physical exercise every single day. The goal with this exercise is not to get rock-hard abs or to lift your butt.

At www.CloseYourEyesLoseWeight.com are diet resources and exercise programs from some of the world's leading experts. But right now, we're not focused on the specific type of movement or even outcome (in terms of sculpting or toning). The goal is to train your brain to love movement until exercise becomes a habit, until you crave exercise. To accomplish this, you must follow an important first step.

> You must overcome the subconscious blocks you have toward exercise so you can rewire your brain to crave a minimum of twenty minutes of exercise, every single day. Once you feel the endorphins, you can stop (although you might not want to).
>
> Step 1: Overcome subconscious blocks to exercising.
> Step 2: Keep moving until you feel the release of endorphins.

---

49 "How Much Exercise Is Necessary for Endorphin Release?," Exercise.com, accessed November 4, 2019, www.exercise.com/learn/how-much-exercise-is-necessary-for-endorphin-release/.

Be Aware of Sneaky Self-Sabotage!

The most common form of self-sabotage I see with clients beginning a new exercise regime is to go too hard, too fast. The subconscious says, "Oh sure, you want to exercise. How about you go for a mile-long run after sitting on your couch every night for the last five years? You played softball in high school. I'm sure you've still got it in you. Come on, didn't you say it's 'new year, new you'? Let's do this!" Then off she goes, jogging at full tilt, with an extra forty-five pounds on the body that weren't there in high school, plus decades of no training in between. And what happens? She's wobbling home with a hurt knee or ankle or back, so much so that after her first or second run, where do you think she's landed? Back on the couch. Taken to the extreme, exercising too hard, too fast can include a hospital stay and painkillers, which can lead to a host of potentially dangerous issues.

It is imperative to your long-term success that you work with a personal trainer or yoga instructor or another physical fitness expert (or even a highly rated app) to create a program that will allow you to increase your strength and durability *over time* so you're not taken out by a self-sabotage injury on day one.

You might be wondering, "Why would the subconscious sabotage my desire to exercise when exercising releases feel-good endorphins and is necessary for human beings to thrive and live longer?" Great question. The subconscious cares more about *protecting* you than anything. Because it takes around twenty minutes for endorphins to be released, the subconscious does not view this as an immediate solution to a perceived threat. It does not see the benefit over its much preferred traditional course of action—staying the same. Also, if the perceived subconscious reward of keeping weight on is still "safer" than the perceived benefits of exercising, Resistance will show up. You have to actively let the subconscious know with conditioning that the endorphins released via exercise **are keeping you safe**. These are the concepts this week's hypnosis recording and self-hypnosis practice will cover.

Once exercise becomes *habitual*, an automatic program running in the background, it's much, much easier to keep it up because you'll be *craving* it. Our work together is to get you from where you are to a daily practice of at least twenty minutes of movement per day, until it becomes habitual. Until you love it. Until you crave it. Pop in those headphones, and let's get to work!

Homework

A. Practice self-hypnosis three times a day, every day this week (right before breakfast, lunch, and dinner). Turn to page 20 for a reminder of how to do self-hypnosis or head to www. CloseYourEyesLoseWeight.com to follow along with a tutorial video.

Week 4 Hypno-affirmations—Exercise

- Every day in every way I move my body until I feel those amazing endorphins for at least twenty minutes.
- I love to exercise.
- I crave exercising.
- When I exercise for twenty minutes, I feel so happy.
- My body craves movement.
- Every day in every way I get my heart rate up for at least twenty minutes.

B. Listen to the "Week 4—Exercise" hypnosis recording every day for the next week here: www.CloseYourEyesLoseWeight.com.

C. Use your journal pages daily to stay motivated, log your progress, and determine which pick-me-up hypno-affirmations you'll benefit from most.

. . . .

You're really doing this. Exercise is *amazing*, isn't it? You crave movement every single day because you know just how good those endorphins are going to feel. Great job! In the next chapter, you'll learn a powerful process to help you get to the root of one of the greatest detractors of weight loss success . . . emotional eating. Turn the page and let's get started!

WEEK 4 LOG

TRACK YOUR PROGRESS

TODAY

Weight	Measurements		How Do You Feel in Your Clothes?	What's Your Energy Level?
	Neck:	Waist:		
	Chest:	Hips:	1 2 3 4 5	1 2 3 4 5
	(L) Arm	(L) Thigh:		
	(R) Arm	(R) Thigh:		

Write down any negative thoughts, immediately cross them out, and replace them with a positive thought.

CANCEL-CANCEL BOX

··

[PRO TIP] Stay neutral. Get curious!

··

How Will You Conjure Up Additional Energy When Needed?

10 jumping jacks ___   Shout hypno-affirmations ___   Other ___

Water

8oz of water before breakfast ___   8oz of water before lunch ___   8oz of water before dinner ___

This Morning's Self-Hypnosis | Round 1: Week 4—Exercise

Time you start: _____   Starting Stress Level (0–10): _____   Ending Stress Level (0–10): _____

This Afternoon's Self-Hypnosis | Round 2: Week 4—Exercise

Time you start: _____   Starting Stress Level (0–10): _____   Ending Stress Level (0–10): _____

This Evening's Self-Hypnosis | Round 3: Week 4—Exercise

Time you start: _____   Starting Stress Level (0–10): _____   Ending Stress Level (0–10): _____

Listen to this week's assigned hypnotherapy recording (found at www.CloseYourEyesLoseWeight.com): ☐

Tomorrow's Meal Planning

Breakfast	Snack	Lunch	Snack	Dinner

Check here when tomorrow's meals have been made or ordered: ☐

Visit www.CloseYourEyesLoseWeight.com and share your wins with our community: ☐

WEEK 4 LOG

TRACK YOUR PROGRESS

TODAY

Weight	Measurements	How Do You Feel in Your Clothes?	What's Your Energy Level?
	Neck: Waist:		
	Chest: Hips:	1 2 3 4 5	1 2 3 4 5
	(L) Arm (L) Thigh:		
	(R) Arm (R) Thigh:		

Write down any negative thoughts, immediately cross them out, and replace them with a positive thought.

CANCEL-CANCEL BOX

[PRO TIP] Stay neutral. Get curious!

How Will You Conjure Up Additional Energy When Needed?

10 jumping jacks ___   Shout hypno-affirmations ___   Other ___

Water

8oz of water before breakfast ___   8oz of water before lunch ___   8oz of water before dinner ___

This Morning's Self-Hypnosis | Round 1: Week 4—Exercise

Time you start: _____   Starting Stress Level (0–10): _____   Ending Stress Level (0–10): _____

This Afternoon's Self-Hypnosis | Round 2: Week 4—Exercise

Time you start: _____   Starting Stress Level (0–10): _____   Ending Stress Level (0–10): _____

This Evening's Self-Hypnosis | Round 3: Week 4—Exercise

Time you start: _____   Starting Stress Level (0–10): _____   Ending Stress Level (0–10): _____

Listen to this week's assigned hypnotherapy recording (found at www.CloseYourEyesLoseWeight.com): ☐

Tomorrow's Meal Planning

Breakfast	Snack	Lunch	Snack	Dinner

Check here when tomorrow's meals have been made or ordered: ☐

Visit www.CloseYourEyesLoseWeight.com and share your wins with our community: ☐

WEEK 4 LOG

TRACK YOUR PROGRESS

TODAY

Weight	Measurements	How Do You Feel in Your Clothes?	What's Your Energy Level?
	Neck: Waist:		
	Chest: Hips:		
	(L) Arm (L) Thigh:	1 2 3 4 5	1 2 3 4 5
	(R) Arm (R) Thigh:		

Write down any negative thoughts, immediately cross them out, and replace them with a positive thought.

CANCEL-CANCEL BOX

[PRO TIP] Stay neutral. Get curious!

How Will You Conjure Up Additional Energy When Needed?

10 jumping jacks ___   Shout hypno-affirmations ___   Other ___

Water

8oz of water before breakfast ___   8oz of water before lunch ___   8oz of water before dinner ___

This Morning's Self-Hypnosis | Round 1: Week 4—Exercise

Time you start: _____   Starting Stress Level (0–10): _____   Ending Stress Level (0–10): _____

This Afternoon's Self-Hypnosis | Round 2: Week 4—Exercise

Time you start: _____   Starting Stress Level (0–10): _____   Ending Stress Level (0–10): _____

This Evening's Self-Hypnosis | Round 3: Week 4—Exercise

Time you start: _____   Starting Stress Level (0–10): _____   Ending Stress Level (0–10): _____

Listen to this week's assigned hypnotherapy recording (found at www.CloseYourEyesLoseWeight.com): ☐

Tomorrow's Meal Planning

Breakfast	Snack	Lunch	Snack	Dinner

Check here when tomorrow's meals have been made or ordered: ☐

Visit www.CloseYourEyesLoseWeight.com and share your wins with our community: ☐

WEEK 4 LOG

TRACK YOUR PROGRESS

TODAY

Weight	Measurements	How Do You Feel in Your Clothes?	What's Your Energy Level?
	Neck: Waist:		
	Chest: Hips:		
	(L) Arm (L) Thigh:	1 2 3 4 5	1 2 3 4 5
	(R) Arm (R) Thigh:		

Write down any negative thoughts, immediately cross them out, and replace them with a positive thought.

CANCEL-CANCEL BOX

. . . .

[PRO TIP] Stay neutral. Get curious!

. . . .

How Will You Conjure Up Additional Energy When Needed?

10 jumping jacks __   Shout hypno-affirmations __   Other __

Water

8oz of water before breakfast __   8oz of water before lunch __   8oz of water before dinner __

This Morning's Self-Hypnosis | Round 1: Week 4—Exercise

Time you start: _____   Starting Stress Level (0–10): _____   Ending Stress Level (0–10): _____

This Afternoon's Self-Hypnosis | Round 2: Week 4—Exercise

Time you start: _____   Starting Stress Level (0–10): _____   Ending Stress Level (0–10): _____

This Evening's Self-Hypnosis | Round 3: Week 4—Exercise

Time you start: _____   Starting Stress Level (0–10): _____   Ending Stress Level (0–10): _____

Listen to this week's assigned hypnotherapy recording (found at www.CloseYourEyesLoseWeight.com): ☐

Tomorrow's Meal Planning

Breakfast	Snack	Lunch	Snack	Dinner

Check here when tomorrow's meals have been made or ordered: ☐

Visit www.CloseYourEyesLoseWeight.com and share your wins with our community: ☐

TRACK YOUR PROGRESS

TODAY

Weight	Measurements	How Do You Feel in Your Clothes?	What's Your Energy Level?
	Neck: Waist:		
	Chest: Hips:	1 2 3 4 5	1 2 3 4 5
	(L) Arm (L) Thigh:		
	(R) Arm (R) Thigh:		

Write down any negative thoughts, immediately cross them out, and replace them with a positive thought.

CANCEL-CANCEL BOX

[PRO TIP] Stay neutral. Get curious!

How Will You Conjure Up Additional Energy When Needed?

10 jumping jacks ___   Shout hypno-affirmations ___   Other ___

Water

8oz of water before breakfast ___   8oz of water before lunch ___   8oz of water before dinner ___

This Morning's Self-Hypnosis | Round 1: Week 4—Exercise

Time you start: _____   Starting Stress Level (0-10): _____   Ending Stress Level (0-10): _____

This Afternoon's Self-Hypnosis | Round 2: Week 4—Exercise

Time you start: _____   Starting Stress Level (0-10): _____   Ending Stress Level (0-10): _____

This Evening's Self-Hypnosis | Round 3: Week 4—Exercise

Time you start: _____   Starting Stress Level (0-10): _____   Ending Stress Level (0-10): _____

Listen to this week's assigned hypnotherapy recording (found at www.CloseYourEyesLoseWeight.com): ☐

Tomorrow's Meal Planning

Breakfast	Snack	Lunch	Snack	Dinner

Check here when tomorrow's meals have been made or ordered: ☐

Visit www.CloseYourEyesLoseWeight.com and share your wins with our community: ☐

WEEK 4 LOG

TRACK YOUR PROGRESS

TODAY

Weight	Measurements	How Do You Feel in Your Clothes?	What's Your Energy Level?
	Neck: Waist:		
	Chest: Hips:	1 2 3 4 5	1 2 3 4 5
	(L) Arm (L) Thigh:		
	(R) Arm (R) Thigh:		

Write down any negative thoughts, immediately cross them out, and replace them with a positive thought.

CANCEL-CANCEL BOX

[PRO TIP] Stay neutral. Get curious!

How Will You Conjure Up Additional Energy When Needed?

10 jumping jacks ___   Shout hypno-affirmations ___   Other ___

Water

8oz of water before breakfast ___   8oz of water before lunch ___   8oz of water before dinner ___

This Morning's Self-Hypnosis | Round 1: Week 4—Exercise

Time you start: _____   Starting Stress Level (0–10): _____   Ending Stress Level (0–10): _____

This Afternoon's Self-Hypnosis | Round 2: Week 4—Exercise

Time you start: _____   Starting Stress Level (0–10): _____   Ending Stress Level (0–10): _____

This Evening's Self-Hypnosis | Round 3: Week 4—Exercise

Time you start: _____   Starting Stress Level (0–10): _____   Ending Stress Level (0–10): _____

Listen to this week's assigned hypnotherapy recording (found at www.CloseYourEyesLoseWeight.com): ☐

Tomorrow's Meal Planning

Breakfast	Snack	Lunch	Snack	Dinner

Check here when tomorrow's meals have been made or ordered: ☐

Visit www.CloseYourEyesLoseWeight.com and share your wins with our community: ☐

WEEK 4 LOG

TRACK YOUR PROGRESS

TODAY

Weight	Measurements	How Do You Feel in Your Clothes?	What's Your Energy Level?
	Neck: Waist:		
	Chest: Hips:	1 2 3 4 5	1 2 3 4 5
	(L) Arm (L) Thigh:		
	(R) Arm (R) Thigh:		

Write down any negative thoughts, immediately cross them out, and replace them with a positive thought.

CANCEL-CANCEL BOX

[PRO TIP] Stay neutral. Get curious!

How Will You Conjure Up Additional Energy When Needed?

10 jumping jacks ___   Shout hypno-affirmations ___   Other ___

Water

8oz of water before breakfast ___   8oz of water before lunch ___   8oz of water before dinner ___

This Morning's Self-Hypnosis | Round 1: Week 4—Exercise

Time you start: _____   Starting Stress Level (0–10): _____   Ending Stress Level (0–10): _____

This Afternoon's Self-Hypnosis | Round 2: Week 4—Exercise

Time you start: _____   Starting Stress Level (0–10): _____   Ending Stress Level (0–10): _____

This Evening's Self-Hypnosis | Round 3: Week 4—Exercise

Time you start: _____   Starting Stress Level (0–10): _____   Ending Stress Level (0–10): _____

Listen to this week's assigned hypnotherapy recording (found at www.CloseYourEyesLoseWeight.com): ☐

Tomorrow's Meal Planning

Breakfast	Snack	Lunch	Snack	Dinner

Check here when tomorrow's meals have been made or ordered: ☐

Visit www.CloseYourEyesLoseWeight.com and share your wins with our community: ☐

PART III

· ·

Weeks 5–8

Progress Tracker

POUNDS LOST

Starting Weight _____

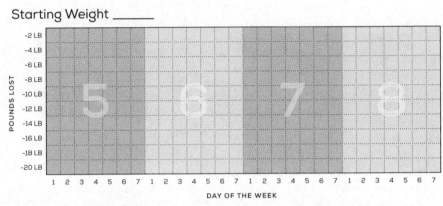

HOW DO YOU FEEL IN YOUR CLOTHES ?

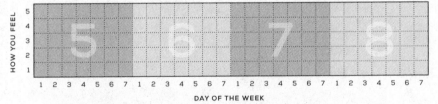

WHAT'S YOUR ENERGY LEVEL?

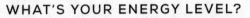
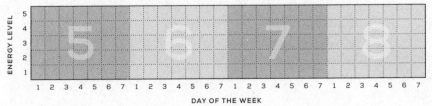

Starting Waist Measurement _____

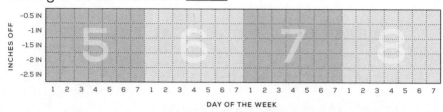

Starting Thigh (L) Measurement _____

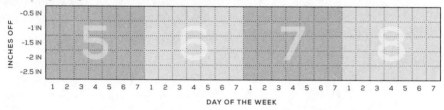

Starting Thigh (R) Measurement _____

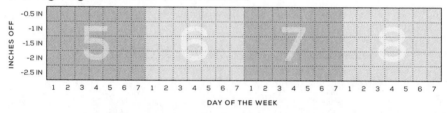

Starting Neck Measurement _____

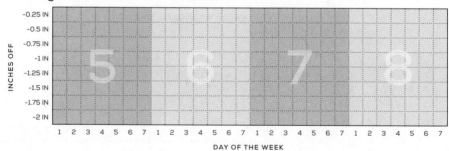

Starting Hip Measurement _____

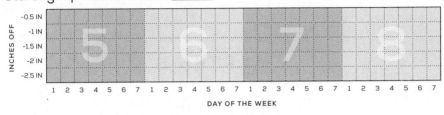

Starting Arm (L) Measurement _____

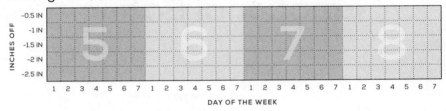

Starting Arm (R) Measurement _____

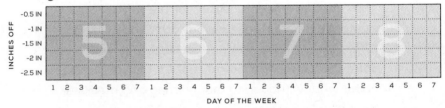

Starting Chest Measurement _____

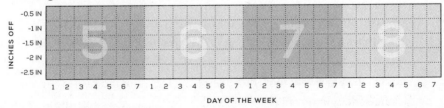

CHAPTER 8

· · · · · · · · · · · · · · · · · · ·

Week 5—
Emotional Eating

> "Junk food has been an issue for me forever. After the first hypnotherapy session with Grace, I began to see my craving thought process interrupted. I don't just jump into a box of cookies. Instead, I think about what is triggering that craving and meditate through it." —Stevonna J., St. Louis, Missouri

You've completed a third of your twelve-week journey, congratulations!

This week is all about learning to "feel your feelings." Emotions are not to be avoided. Nobody likes negative feelings. It's no wonder we drown them out with food, drugs, alcohol, or sex. But these go-to tension relievers don't banish uncomfortable emotions—they bury them.

As we discussed in chapter five, the most common subconscious limiting belief was, "I'm not good enough." If you notice this thought arising, remember that your emotions are a guidance system. When you feel unhappy, sad, not good enough, the emotion wants to tell you something. It's getting your attention. Something is out of alignment.

Oftentimes, though, before the negative thought or emotion has even registered, there's already food in that person's mouth. In this week's hypnosis recording, you're going to learn to become hyperaware of your feelings *before* there's time for emotional eating to begin. If you notice a negative feeling, sit back and observe it. You're not sad. Your body is *experiencing* a sad feeling for a fleeting moment, and that sad feeling wants you to become aware of something. You are the one witnessing the fact that the body is experiencing sadness. You are the *observer*. Take a nice, deep letting-go breath and ask it, "Sad feeling, what do you want to tell me?" You might be surprised at the answer you receive.

Here's an example that might resonate with you: Katie once found herself at a coffee shop eyeing a cheese Danish, something she knew, if she ate it, would taste delicious for a fleeting moment and then she'd feel foggy, bloated, and guilty. Before ordering, she took a deep breath and asked herself the questions she'd learned from her hypnotherapist:

Round 1
Question: Why am I even considering that cheese Danish?
Answer: Because I'm experiencing sadness.

Round 2
Question: Why am I experiencing sadness?
Answer: Because I'm worried that by working on my presentation slides today alone in my hotel room, instead of participating at the conference downstairs, that I'm being left out.

Round 3

Question: Why am I worried about being left out?

Answer: I'm worried people might be talking about me and that they might not like me, or that maybe during the last breakout session I said something stupid and offended someone or made them think less of me. I feel like maybe I should stop working on the presentation slides and go out there so I can try to make a better impression so they won't go home thinking so little of me.

Round 4

Question: Why am I worried that people think so little of me?

Answer: Because in elementary and middle school I was left out and bullied.

Round 5

Question: How did that make me feel?

Answer: Awful.

Round 6

Question: Why did it make me feel awful?

Answer: Because it meant I wasn't good enough to hang out with them.

Round 7

Question: How did that make me feel?

Answer: Lonely.

Round 8

Question: Why did it make me feel lonely?

Answer: Because if I wasn't good enough to hang out with them, I'd never have girlfriends and I'd always be lonely or an outcast.

Conclusion 1

Question: What unhelpful belief did I come to believe about this situation?

Answer: That I can't trust women to not make fun of me, that they don't like me, that I'm not good enough to be their friend.

Conclusion 2

Question: How would I like to feel instead?

Answer: Calm, confident, and focused.

Conclusion 3

Question: What would I like to do instead?

Answer: Continue working on this presentation for now (free from guilt or worry) and get back out there to meet interesting new people at the gala tonight where I will ask questions and provide support rather than talking about myself.

Conclusion 4

Question: What would I like to eat instead?

Answer: Nothing. I just want some water and to continue working.

We could keep going, but you can see how Katie realized that the cheese Danish had more to do with the fact that in fifth grade she walked into a room full of girls pointing and laughing at a photo of her "eight-head" (as opposed to "forehead") in the school yearbook, and as a result her subconscious made her believe she wasn't pretty enough, or good enough to be friends with the cool girls. Even more literally, that her forehead wasn't small enough for her to be liked or accepted. In fact, up until that moment, it made Katie believe she couldn't trust women not to make fun of her. Interestingly enough, in adulthood most of her subconscious limitations revolved around wanting to make sure people liked her.

Isn't it amazing that all this deep wounding was uncovered through such a simple process, simply asking a few questions when triggered to eat something unhelpful? Deep childhood pain had been triggered by the day's events, and in the body's frantic attempt to feel better, it decided a cheese Danish would provide the dopamine hit followed by a sugar-gluten-dairy-induced foggy haze that could momentarily quell all the uncomfortable (read: unsafe) feelings. It might sound silly, but this is a real example of what happens when you dig into the many layers beneath the trigger of emotional eating.

Once Katie took a moment to unpack all of that, do you think she wanted the cheese Danish? Of course not. In fact, by the time she got to "because in elementary school I was left out," she didn't want it anymore, and the sadness was already dissipating. By facing things that were once buried, they lose their power. By bringing our shadows into the light, they begin to disappear. Katie's adult self can look back at that experience in fifth grade and say, "Huh, I didn't realize that was still in there or that it's still affecting me so deeply. I'll put this on my list to work on during my next hypnotherapy session," then make a helpful choice by drinking water, forgetting the cheese Danish, and getting back to work.

Now you're going to learn how to do this practice for yourself. Notice how Katie switched the question from "why" to "how did that make me feel" during round five. Imagine she had asked, "Why did the girls make fun of me?" The answer would have been, "Because I have a big forehead." Short of surgery or a perpetual haircut with bangs, she would have been stuck . . . There's not a solution there. Or she could have said, "Because the girls were mean." But where does she go from there?

Why were they mean? Because people were mean to them or because the other girls were being mean and they didn't want to be ostracized for not participating. Sure, Katie could cultivate compassion for the root cause of *their* issue, but it wouldn't get to the root of *her* issue. We formulate the questions in such a way that you get to the root of *your* issue, not anyone else's (even if you wanted to, you couldn't fix their stuff anyway . . . for that to happen, they'll need to embark upon their own hypnotherapy journey!).

Here are the questions to ask yourself when you find yourself beginning to reach out for that unhelpful food:

Round 1

Why am I even considering eating [insert unhelpful food]?

Answer: _____

Rounds 2 and beyond

Why do I feel [insert answer from round 1]?

Or, How does that make me feel?

Conclusion 1

What unhelpful belief did you come to believe about this situation?

Conclusion 2

How do you want to **feel** instead?

Do one round of self-hypnosis on this now.

Conclusion 3

What do you want to **do** instead?

Take action on this now.

Conclusion 4
What do you want to **eat** instead?

_____

Take action on this now and make sure you chew every bite until only liquid remains!

Think back to the most recent time you went to eat something unhelpful and, with that in mind, take some time to fill out at least one round now.

Homework

A. Practice self-hypnosis three times a day, every day this week (right before breakfast, lunch, and dinner). Turn to page 20 for a reminder of how to do self-hypnosis or head to www. CloseYourEyesLose Weight.com to follow along with a tutorial video.

Week 5 Hypno-affirmations–Emotional Eating

- When I notice myself reaching for unhelpful food, I stop and ask, "What's at the root?"
- I choose to feel _____
  [insert positive emotion] instead.
- When I want to feel better, I use hypnosis to improve my state (instead of food).
- Every day in every way, I ask myself, "Why am I *really* feeling this way?"
- I observe emotions as they come and go. I am watching them. They are separate from me.

- When I feel emotional I stop and say, "I'll only eat what's helpful today."

B. Listen to the "Week 5–Emotional Eating" hypnosis recording every day for the next week here: www. CloseYourEyesLoseWeight.com.

C. Use your journal pages daily to stay motivated, log your progress, and determine which pick-me-up hypno-affirmations you'll benefit from most.

• • • • • • • • • • • • • • • • •

Now that you know how to tackle emotional eating, it's time to address the opposite side of the same coin . . . eating when bored. In the next chapter, you'll learn why boredom eating is the second most common reason weight loss attempts failed in the past. You're going to learn how to wake up from unconscious eating, and how to address the lull of boredom with techniques that don't include food. Cultivate some energy (return to chapter three for tips on how to do this), and let's continue!

WEEK 5 LOG

TRACK YOUR PROGRESS

TODAY

Weight	Measurements	How Do You Feel in Your Clothes?	What's Your Energy Level?
	Neck: Waist:		
	Chest: Hips:	1 2 3 4 5	1 2 3 4 5
	(L) Arm (L) Thigh:		
	(R) Arm (R) Thigh:		

Write down any negative thoughts, immediately cross them out, and replace them with a positive thought.

CANCEL-CANCEL BOX

[PRO TIP] Stay neutral. Get curious!

How Will You Conjure Up Additional Energy When Needed?

10 jumping jacks ___   Shout hypno-affirmations ___   Other ___

Water

8oz of water before breakfast ___   8oz of water before lunch ___   8oz of water before dinner ___

This Morning's Self-Hypnosis | Round 1: Week 5—Emotional Eating

Time you start: _____   Starting Stress Level (0–10): _____   Ending Stress Level (0–10): _____

This Afternoon's Self-Hypnosis | Round 2: Week 5—Emotional Eating

Time you start: _____   Starting Stress Level (0–10): _____   Ending Stress Level (0–10): _____

This Evening's Self-Hypnosis | Round 3: Week 5—Emotional Eating

Time you start: _____   Starting Stress Level (0–10): _____   Ending Stress Level (0–10): _____

Listen to this week's assigned hypnotherapy recording (found at www.CloseYourEyesLoseWeight.com): ☐

Tomorrow's Meal Planning

Breakfast	Snack	Lunch	Snack	Dinner

Check here when tomorrow's meals have been made or ordered: ☐

Visit www.CloseYourEyesLoseWeight.com and share your wins with our community: ☐

WEEK 5 LOG

TRACK YOUR PROGRESS

TODAY

Weight	Measurements	How Do You Feel in Your Clothes?	What's Your Energy Level?
	Neck: Waist:		
	Chest: Hips:	1 2 3 4 5	1 2 3 4 5
	(L) Arm (L) Thigh:		
	(R) Arm (R) Thigh:		

Write down any negative thoughts, immediately cross them out, and replace them with a positive thought.

CANCEL-CANCEL BOX

[PRO TIP] Stay neutral. Get curious!

How Will You Conjure Up Additional Energy When Needed?

10 jumping jacks ___   Shout hypno-affirmations ___   Other ___

Water

8oz of water before breakfast ___   8oz of water before lunch ___   8oz of water before dinner ___

This Morning's Self-Hypnosis | Round 1: Week 5—Emotional Eating

Time you start: _____   Starting Stress Level (0–10): _____   Ending Stress Level (0–10): _____

This Afternoon's Self-Hypnosis | Round 2: Week 5—Emotional Eating

Time you start: _____   Starting Stress Level (0–10): _____   Ending Stress Level (0–10): _____

This Evening's Self-Hypnosis | Round 3: Week 5—Emotional Eating

Time you start: _____   Starting Stress Level (0–10): _____   Ending Stress Level (0–10): _____

Listen to this week's assigned hypnotherapy recording (found at www.CloseYourEyesLoseWeight.com): ☐

Tomorrow's Meal Planning

Breakfast	Snack	Lunch	Snack	Dinner

Check here when tomorrow's meals have been made or ordered: ☐

Visit www.CloseYourEyesLoseWeight.com and share your wins with our community: ☐

TRACK YOUR PROGRESS

TODAY

Weight	Measurements	How Do You Feel in Your Clothes?	What's Your Energy Level?
	Neck: Waist:		
	Chest: Hips:	1 2 3 4 5	1 2 3 4 5
	(L) Arm (L) Thigh:		
	(R) Arm (R) Thigh:		

Write down any negative thoughts, immediately cross them out, and replace them with a positive thought.

CANCEL-CANCEL BOX

[PRO TIP] Stay neutral. Get curious!

How Will You Conjure Up Additional Energy When Needed?

10 jumping jacks ___   Shout hypno-affirmations ___   Other ___

Water

8oz of water before breakfast ___   8oz of water before lunch ___   8oz of water before dinner ___

This Morning's Self-Hypnosis | Round 1: Week 5—Emotional Eating

Time you start: _____   Starting Stress Level (0–10): _____   Ending Stress Level (0–10): _____

This Afternoon's Self-Hypnosis | Round 2: Week 5—Emotional Eating

Time you start: _____   Starting Stress Level (0–10): _____   Ending Stress Level (0–10): _____

This Evening's Self-Hypnosis | Round 3: Week 5—Emotional Eating

Time you start: _____   Starting Stress Level (0–10): _____   Ending Stress Level (0–10): _____

Listen to this week's assigned hypnotherapy recording (found at www.CloseYourEyesLoseWeight.com): ☐

Tomorrow's Meal Planning

Breakfast	Snack	Lunch	Snack	Dinner

Check here when tomorrow's meals have been made or ordered: ☐

Visit www.CloseYourEyesLoseWeight.com and share your wins with our community: ☐

WEEK 5 LOG

DATE: __ / __ / __

TRACK YOUR PROGRESS

TODAY

Weight	Measurements		How Do You Feel in Your Clothes?	What's Your Energy Level?
	Neck:	Waist:		
	Chest:	Hips:	1 2 3 4 5	1 2 3 4 5
	(L) Arm	(L) Thigh:		
	(R) Arm	(R) Thigh:		

Write down any negative thoughts, immediately cross them out, and replace them with a positive thought.

CANCEL-CANCEL BOX

[PRO TIP] Stay neutral. Get curious!

How Will You Conjure Up Additional Energy When Needed?

10 jumping jacks __   Shout hypno-affirmations __   Other __

Water

8oz of water before breakfast __   8oz of water before lunch __   8oz of water before dinner __

This Morning's Self-Hypnosis | Round 1: Week 5—Emotional Eating

Time you start: _____   Starting Stress Level (0–10): _____   Ending Stress Level (0–10): _____

This Afternoon's Self-Hypnosis | Round 2: Week 5—Emotional Eating

Time you start: _____   Starting Stress Level (0–10): _____   Ending Stress Level (0–10): _____

This Evening's Self-Hypnosis | Round 3: Week 5—Emotional Eating

Time you start: _____   Starting Stress Level (0–10): _____   Ending Stress Level (0–10): _____

Listen to this week's assigned hypnotherapy recording (found at www.CloseYourEyesLoseWeight.com): ☐

Tomorrow's Meal Planning

Breakfast	Snack	Lunch	Snack	Dinner

Check here when tomorrow's meals have been made or ordered: ☐

Visit www.CloseYourEyesLoseWeight.com and share your wins with our community: ☐

WEEK 5 LOG

TRACK YOUR PROGRESS

TODAY

Weight	Measurements		How Do You Feel in Your Clothes?	What's Your Energy Level?
	Neck:	Waist:		
	Chest:	Hips:		
	(L) Arm	(L) Thigh:	1 2 3 4 5	1 2 3 4 5
	(R) Arm	(R) Thigh:		

Write down any negative thoughts, immediately cross them out, and replace them with a positive thought.

CANCEL-CANCEL BOX

[PRO TIP] Stay neutral. Get curious!

How Will You Conjure Up Additional Energy When Needed?

10 jumping jacks ___   Shout hypno-affirmations ___   Other ___

Water

8oz of water before breakfast ___   8oz of water before lunch ___   8oz of water before dinner ___

This Morning's Self-Hypnosis | Round 1: Week 5–Emotional Eating

Time you start: _____   Starting Stress Level (0–10): _____   Ending Stress Level (0–10): _____

This Afternoon's Self-Hypnosis | Round 2: Week 5–Emotional Eating

Time you start: _____   Starting Stress Level (0–10): _____   Ending Stress Level (0–10): _____

This Evening's Self-Hypnosis | Round 3: Week 5–Emotional Eating

Time you start: _____   Starting Stress Level (0–10): _____   Ending Stress Level (0–10): _____

Listen to this week's assigned hypnotherapy recording (found at www.CloseYourEyesLoseWeight.com): ☐

Tomorrow's Meal Planning

Breakfast	Snack	Lunch	Snack	Dinner

Check here when tomorrow's meals have been made or ordered: ☐

Visit www.CloseYourEyesLoseWeight.com and share your wins with our community: ☐

WEEK 5 LOG

TRACK YOUR PROGRESS

TODAY

Weight	Measurements	How Do You Feel in Your Clothes?	What's Your Energy Level?
	Neck: Waist:		
	Chest: Hips:		
	(L) Arm (L) Thigh:	1 2 3 4 5	1 2 3 4 5
	(R) Arm (R) Thigh:		

Write down any negative thoughts, immediately cross them out, and replace them with a positive thought.

CANCEL-CANCEL BOX

[PRO TIP] Stay neutral. Get curious!

How Will You Conjure Up Additional Energy When Needed?

10 jumping jacks ___   Shout hypno-affirmations ___   Other ___

Water

8oz of water before breakfast ___   8oz of water before lunch ___   8oz of water before dinner ___

This Morning's Self-Hypnosis | Round 1: Week 5—Emotional Eating

Time you start: _____   Starting Stress Level (0–10): _____   Ending Stress Level (0–10): _____

This Afternoon's Self-Hypnosis | Round 2: Week 5—Emotional Eating

Time you start: _____   Starting Stress Level (0–10): _____   Ending Stress Level (0–10): _____

This Evening's Self-Hypnosis | Round 3: Week 5—Emotional Eating

Time you start: _____   Starting Stress Level (0–10): _____   Ending Stress Level (0–10): _____

Listen to this week's assigned hypnotherapy recording (found at www.CloseYourEyesLoseWeight.com): ☐

Tomorrow's Meal Planning

Breakfast	Snack	Lunch	Snack	Dinner

Check here when tomorrow's meals have been made or ordered: ☐

Visit www.CloseYourEyesLoseWeight.com and share your wins with our community: ☐

WEEK 5 LOG

TRACK YOUR PROGRESS

TODAY

Weight	Measurements	How Do You Feel in Your Clothes?	What's Your Energy Level?
	Neck: Waist:		
	Chest: Hips:	1 2 3 4 5	1 2 3 4 5
	(L) Arm (L) Thigh:		
	(R) Arm (R) Thigh:		

Write down any negative thoughts, immediately cross them out, and replace them with a positive thought.

CANCEL-CANCEL BOX

[PRO TIP] Stay neutral. Get curious!

How Will You Conjure Up Additional Energy When Needed?

10 jumping jacks ___   Shout hypno-affirmations ___   Other ___

Water

8oz of water before breakfast ___   8oz of water before lunch ___   8oz of water before dinner ___

This Morning's Self-Hypnosis | Round 1: Week 5—Emotional Eating

Time you start: _____   Starting Stress Level (0–10): _____   Ending Stress Level (0–10): _____

This Afternoon's Self-Hypnosis | Round 2: Week 5—Emotional Eating

Time you start: _____   Starting Stress Level (0–10): _____   Ending Stress Level (0–10): _____

This Evening's Self-Hypnosis | Round 3: Week 5—Emotional Eating

Time you start: _____   Starting Stress Level (0–10): _____   Ending Stress Level (0–10): _____

Listen to this week's assigned hypnotherapy recording (found at www.CloseYourEyesLoseWeight.com): ☐

Tomorrow's Meal Planning

Breakfast	Snack	Lunch	Snack	Dinner

Check here when tomorrow's meals have been made or ordered: ☐

Visit www.CloseYourEyesLoseWeight.com and share your wins with our community: ☐

CHAPTER 9

· · · · · · · · · · · · ·

Week 6– Eating When Bored

"I used to say, 'There's nothing to do. I'm bored, I don't have the energy to go for a walk, read a book, start a new hobby. I feel depressed about that, so I go digging for food and I sit on the couch, zone out, and eat mindlessly from a bag of chips. I feel better, even if only momentarily.' This cycle would have continued forever if I hadn't reprogrammed my subconscious mind. I'm so grateful I did. I not only no longer eat when I'm bored, I rarely ever feel bored in the first place." –Marc L., London, England

After emotional eating, eating when bored is the second biggest impediment to weight loss. When you're bored, you are *not* feeling exhilaration, happiness, or excitement. In fact, extended boredom can feel like depression. In the same way that we eat to change our emotional state, we eat to snap out of boredom, a state devoid of emotions altogether.

There's nothing like dopamine to perk you up, even if a quick hit crashes you lower than where you started. Dopamine is a neurotransmitter in the brain that plays a major role in reward-motivated behavior. To put it simply, dopamine is the brain's "desire" chemical associated with the feeling you get when achieving a goal.

As mentioned in chapter one, specific foods contribute to an increase in dopamine levels. These foods are generally categorized as "junk food"—those high in sugar, fat, and sodium content. Foods like these cause the body to release endorphins, aka feel-good hormones. It's safe to assume that when you're bored, you aren't reaching for that plate of brussels sprouts. A series of studies by researchers at the University of Limerick, Ireland, indicate that "boredom increases eating, specifically unhealthy and exciting foods which can serve as means to escape the bored self."[50]

The real challenge here is that eating *does* make us feel better when we're bored. That's not made up—it's real. According to an article in *Psychology Today*,

> It's possible that when we're in a malaise, so are our dopamine neurons. When we boredom-eat what we're really doing is trying to wake them up so we can feel excited again . . . After all, our dopamine system evolved with the very purpose of making adaptive things like eating feel rewarding, so that we wouldn't forget to do them and die. And one survey study recently found that

---

50 Andrew B. Moynihan et al., "Eaten Up by Boredom: Consuming Food to Escape Awareness of the Bored Self," *Frontiers in Psychology* 6 (2015), http://ncbi. nlm.nih.gov/pmc/articles/PMC4381486/.

the happiest moments of a typical participant's day were
the ones where he or she was eating something.[51]

While eating triggering food may make us feel better in the
short term, over time those same foods can wreak havoc on our
health. The solution is to retrain the subconscious to choose what is
uncomfortable in the short term (now) but wonderful in the long
term. In all areas of life, and especially when it comes to weight
loss, we benefit from programming our minds to choose long-term
growth over short-term pleasure.

Evaluating the deeper reasoning behind the boredom and developing proactive ways to break out of it will help, as will learning to
wake up from this trance of boredom eating. As you might be starting to recognize, with hypnotherapy you're actually de-hypnotizing
yourself. There are three main antidotes to eating when bored:

1. Become consciously aware of the fact that you're
   eating (since most boredom eating is unconscious).
2. Learn new ways of dealing with boredom.
3. Over time, train yourself to take different actions
   altogether when boredom sets in.

You're going to train yourself to do these three things in this
week's hypnosis recording. You'll become hyperaware of any time
that you're putting food into your mouth ("Cancel, cancel!" mind-
less eating and replace it with mindful eating!) and you'll use tac-
tics similar to what we used during our motivational prep-week

---

51 Susan Carnell, "Do You Eat out of Boredom?," *Psychology Today*, December
4, 2011, www.psychologytoday.com/us/blog/bad-appetite/201112/do-you-eat
-out-boredom.

recording to snap you out of boredom without using food. Here are some other areas you'll cover with this week's hypnosis recording:

- What is boredom covering up for you? In other words, what emotions or thoughts are buried beneath the boredom?
- What are the ways your mind pretends that boredom is keeping you safe? How long has it been doing this?
- What massive breakthroughs could you experience by facing what's buried beneath boredom and working on the root issue?

There are some interesting answers beneath those layers of protective self-sabotage, which, in this instance, are dressed up as boredom. I'll be interested to find out what you uncover!

Homework

A. Practice self-hypnosis three times a day, every day this week (right before breakfast, lunch, and dinner). Turn to page 20 for a reminder of how to do self-hypnosis or head to www. CloseYourEyesLoseWeight.com to follow along with a tutorial video.

Week 6 Hypno-affirmations—Eating When Bored

- Every day in every way I am more and more aware of everything I eat.
- I choose to eat mindfully with awareness.

- When I eat, I eat. That's it.
- When I eat, I focus on the taste of the food as I chew until only liquid remains. That is all.
- I am awake and alert when I eat.
- For a boost of energy, I jump up and down and change my state.

B. Listen to the "Week 6—Eating When Bored" hypnosis recording every day for the next week here: www.CloseYourEyesLoseWeight.com.

C. Use your journal pages daily to stay motivated, log your progress, and determine which pick-me-up hypno-affirmations you'll benefit from most.

. . . .

Boredom has been broken! You're free to live an exciting, energizing life. As for what you'll learn in chapter ten, it's simple. No more rewarding yourself with "poison"—it's time to reward yourself with health and vitality. Turn the page, and let's get to it!

TRACK YOUR PROGRESS

TODAY

Weight	Measurements	How Do You Feel in Your Clothes?	What's Your Energy Level?
	Neck: Waist:		
	Chest: Hips:	1 2 3 4 5	1 2 3 4 5
	(L) Arm (L) Thigh:		
	(R) Arm (R) Thigh:		

Write down any negative thoughts, immediately cross them out, and replace them with a positive thought.

CANCEL-CANCEL BOX

[PRO TIP] Stay neutral. Get curious!

How Will You Conjure Up Additional Energy When Needed?

10 jumping jacks ___   Shout hypno-affirmations ___   Other ___

Water

8oz of water before breakfast ___   8oz of water before lunch ___   8oz of water before dinner ___

This Morning's Self-Hypnosis | Round 1: Week 6—Eating When Bored

Time you start: _____   Starting Stress Level (0–10): _____   Ending Stress Level (0–10): _____

This Afternoon's Self-Hypnosis | Round 2: Week 6—Eating When Bored

Time you start: _____   Starting Stress Level (0–10): _____   Ending Stress Level (0–10): _____

This Evening's Self-Hypnosis | Round 3: Week 6—Eating When Bored

Time you start: _____   Starting Stress Level (0–10): _____   Ending Stress Level (0–10): _____

Listen to this week's assigned hypnotherapy recording (found at www.CloseYourEyesLoseWeight.com): ☐

Tomorrow's Meal Planning

Breakfast	Snack	Lunch	Snack	Dinner

Check here when tomorrow's meals have been made or ordered: ☐

Visit www.CloseYourEyesLoseWeight.com and share your wins with our community: ☐

WEEK 6 LOG

TRACK YOUR PROGRESS

TODAY	Weight	Measurements		How Do You Feel in Your Clothes?	What's Your Energy Level?
		Neck:	Waist:		
		Chest:	Hips:		
		(L) Arm	(L) Thigh:	1 2 3 4 5	1 2 3 4 5
		(R) Arm	(R) Thigh:		

Write down any negative thoughts, immediately cross them out, and replace them with a positive thought.

CANCEL-CANCEL BOX

[PRO TIP] Stay neutral. Get curious!

How Will You Conjure Up Additional Energy When Needed?

10 jumping jacks ___   Shout hypno-affirmations ___   Other ___

Water

8oz of water before breakfast ___   8oz of water before lunch ___   8oz of water before dinner ___

This Morning's Self-Hypnosis | Round 1: Week 6–Eating When Bored

Time you start: _____   Starting Stress Level (0–10): _____   Ending Stress Level (0–10): _____

This Afternoon's Self-Hypnosis | Round 2: Week 6–Eating When Bored

Time you start: _____   Starting Stress Level (0–10): _____   Ending Stress Level (0–10): _____

This Evening's Self-Hypnosis | Round 3: Week 6–Eating When Bored

Time you start: _____   Starting Stress Level (0–10): _____   Ending Stress Level (0–10): _____

Listen to this week's assigned hypnotherapy recording (found at www.CloseYourEyesLoseWeight.com): ☐

Tomorrow's Meal Planning

Breakfast	Snack	Lunch	Snack	Dinner

Check here when tomorrow's meals have been made or ordered: ☐

Visit www.CloseYourEyesLoseWeight.com and share your wins with our community: ☐

WEEK 6 LOG

TRACK YOUR PROGRESS

TODAY

Weight	Measurements		How Do You Feel in Your Clothes?	What's Your Energy Level?
	Neck:	Waist:		
	Chest:	Hips:		
	(L) Arm	(L) Thigh:	1 2 3 4 5	1 2 3 4 5
	(R) Arm	(R) Thigh:		

Write down any negative thoughts, immediately cross them out, and replace them with a positive thought.

CANCEL-CANCEL BOX

[PRO TIP] Stay neutral. Get curious!

How Will You Conjure Up Additional Energy When Needed?

10 jumping jacks ___   Shout hypno-affirmations ___   Other ___

Water

8oz of water before breakfast ___   8oz of water before lunch ___   8oz of water before dinner ___

This Morning's Self-Hypnosis | Round 1: Week 6—Eating When Bored

Time you start: _____   Starting Stress Level (0–10): _____   Ending Stress Level (0–10): _____

This Afternoon's Self-Hypnosis | Round 2: Week 6—Eating When Bored

Time you start: _____   Starting Stress Level (0–10): _____   Ending Stress Level (0–10): _____

This Evening's Self-Hypnosis | Round 3: Week 6—Eating When Bored

Time you start: _____   Starting Stress Level (0–10): _____   Ending Stress Level (0–10): _____

Listen to this week's assigned hypnotherapy recording (found at www.CloseYourEyesLoseWeight.com): ☐

Tomorrow's Meal Planning

Breakfast	Snack	Lunch	Snack	Dinner

Check here when tomorrow's meals have been made or ordered: ☐

Visit www.CloseYourEyesLoseWeight.com and share your wins with our community: ☐

TRACK YOUR PROGRESS

TODAY

Weight	Measurements	How Do You Feel in Your Clothes?	What's Your Energy Level?
	Neck: Waist:		
	Chest: Hips:	1 2 3 4 5	1 2 3 4 5
	(L) Arm (L) Thigh:		
	(R) Arm (R) Thigh:		

Write down any negative thoughts, immediately cross them out, and replace them with a positive thought.

CANCEL-CANCEL BOX

[PRO TIP] Stay neutral. Get curious!

How Will You Conjure Up Additional Energy When Needed?

10 jumping jacks ___   Shout hypno-affirmations ___   Other ___

Water

8oz of water before breakfast ___   8oz of water before lunch ___   8oz of water before dinner ___

This Morning's Self-Hypnosis | Round 1: Week 6—Eating When Bored

Time you start: _____   Starting Stress Level (0–10): _____   Ending Stress Level (0–10): _____

This Afternoon's Self-Hypnosis | Round 2: Week 6—Eating When Bored

Time you start: _____   Starting Stress Level (0–10): _____   Ending Stress Level (0–10): _____

This Evening's Self-Hypnosis | Round 3: Week 6—Eating When Bored

Time you start: _____   Starting Stress Level (0–10): _____   Ending Stress Level (0–10): _____

Listen to this week's assigned hypnotherapy recording (found at www.CloseYourEyesLoseWeight.com): ☐

Tomorrow's Meal Planning

Breakfast	Snack	Lunch	Snack	Dinner

Check here when tomorrow's meals have been made or ordered: ☐

Visit www.CloseYourEyesLoseWeight.com and share your wins with our community: ☐

WEEK 6 LOG

TRACK YOUR PROGRESS

TODAY

Weight	Measurements	How Do You Feel in Your Clothes?	What's Your Energy Level?
	Neck: ___ Waist: ___		
	Chest: ___ Hips: ___	1 2 3 4 5	1 2 3 4 5
	(L) Arm ___ (L) Thigh: ___		
	(R) Arm ___ (R) Thigh: ___		

Write down any negative thoughts, immediately cross them out, and replace them with a positive thought.

CANCEL-CANCEL BOX

[PRO TIP] Stay neutral. Get curious!

How Will You Conjure Up Additional Energy When Needed?

10 jumping jacks ___   Shout hypno-affirmations ___   Other ___

Water

8oz of water before breakfast ___   8oz of water before lunch ___   8oz of water before dinner ___

This Morning's Self-Hypnosis | Round 1: Week 6–Eating When Bored

Time you start: _____   Starting Stress Level (0–10): _____   Ending Stress Level (0–10): _____

This Afternoon's Self-Hypnosis | Round 2: Week 6–Eating When Bored

Time you start: _____   Starting Stress Level (0–10): _____   Ending Stress Level (0–10): _____

This Evening's Self-Hypnosis | Round 3: Week 6–Eating When Bored

Time you start: _____   Starting Stress Level (0–10): _____   Ending Stress Level (0–10): _____

Listen to this week's assigned hypnotherapy recording (found at www.CloseYourEyesLoseWeight.com): ☐

Tomorrow's Meal Planning

Breakfast	Snack	Lunch	Snack	Dinner

Check here when tomorrow's meals have been made or ordered: ☐

Visit www.CloseYourEyesLoseWeight.com and share your wins with our community: ☐

WEEK 6 LOG

TRACK YOUR PROGRESS

TODAY

Weight	Measurements	How Do You Feel in Your Clothes?	What's Your Energy Level?
	Neck: Waist:		
	Chest: Hips:	1 2 3 4 5	1 2 3 4 5
	(L) Arm (L) Thigh:		
	(R) Arm (R) Thigh:		

Write down any negative thoughts, immediately cross them out, and replace them with a positive thought.

CANCEL-CANCEL BOX

[PRO TIP] Stay neutral. Get curious!

How Will You Conjure Up Additional Energy When Needed?

10 jumping jacks ___   Shout hypno-affirmations ___   Other ___

Water

8oz of water before breakfast ___   8oz of water before lunch ___   8oz of water before dinner ___

This Morning's Self-Hypnosis | Round 1: Week 6—Eating When Bored

Time you start: _____   Starting Stress Level (0–10): _____   Ending Stress Level (0–10): _____

This Afternoon's Self-Hypnosis | Round 2: Week 6—Eating When Bored

Time you start: _____   Starting Stress Level (0–10): _____   Ending Stress Level (0–10): _____

This Evening's Self-Hypnosis | Round 3: Week 6—Eating When Bored

Time you start: _____   Starting Stress Level (0–10): _____   Ending Stress Level (0–10): _____

Listen to this week's assigned hypnotherapy recording (found at www.CloseYourEyesLoseWeight.com): ☐

Tomorrow's Meal Planning

Breakfast	Snack	Lunch	Snack	Dinner

Check here when tomorrow's meals have been made or ordered: ☐

Visit www.CloseYourEyesLoseWeight.com and share your wins with our community: ☐

TRACK YOUR PROGRESS

TODAY

Weight	Measurements	How Do You Feel in Your Clothes?	What's Your Energy Level?
	Neck: Waist:		
	Chest: Hips:	1 2 3 4 5	1 2 3 4 5
	(L) Arm (L) Thigh:		
	(R) Arm (R) Thigh:		

Write down any negative thoughts, immediately cross them out, and replace them with a positive thought.

CANCEL-CANCEL BOX

[PRO TIP] Stay neutral. Get curious!

How Will You Conjure Up Additional Energy When Needed?

10 jumping jacks ___   Shout hypno-affirmations ___   Other ___

Water

8oz of water before breakfast ___   8oz of water before lunch ___   8oz of water before dinner ___

This Morning's Self-Hypnosis | Round 1: Week 6—Eating When Bored

Time you start: _____   Starting Stress Level (0–10): _____   Ending Stress Level (0–10): _____

This Afternoon's Self-Hypnosis | Round 2: Week 6—Eating When Bored

Time you start: _____   Starting Stress Level (0–10): _____   Ending Stress Level (0–10): _____

This Evening's Self-Hypnosis | Round 3: Week 6—Eating When Bored

Time you start: _____   Starting Stress Level (0–10): _____   Ending Stress Level (0–10): _____

Listen to this week's assigned hypnotherapy recording (found at www.CloseYourEyesLoseWeight.com): ☐

Tomorrow's Meal Planning

Breakfast	Snack	Lunch	Snack	Dinner

Check here when tomorrow's meals have been made or ordered: ☐

Visit www.CloseYourEyesLoseWeight.com and share your wins with our community: ☐

CHAPTER 10

· · · · · · · · · · · · · · · · · · ·

Week 7–
Upgrade How You
Reward Yourself

Every single thing that your subconscious does is because it thinks it's helping you to stay alive. It hates change, it loves routine, and it loves its perceived rewards. There are two areas of reward to consider: (1) the reward of the release of dopamine, (2) the **perceived** rewards of behaving in a certain way.

Here is a common example: My client Alice was in her early sixties. She was inexplicably in pain all the time. She didn't have arthritis, she didn't have fibromyalgia, she didn't have celiac disease. She had been tested for everything under the sun, and her doctors put her on pain medication with no real diagnosis. Alice ached with genuine pain all day, every day. When I asked her conscious mind during our first consultation, "What are all the reasons why you want to get rid of this pain?" her laundry list was a mile long.

"So I can garden, feel better, stop taking these pills, go for walks, play with my grandkids, stop worrying my family, live pain-free, cook, read or watch TV while focusing on the plot."

When I asked Alice's conscious mind what are all the reasons for why she would *want* to hold on to the pain, she looked at me incredulously and said, "There is not one reason why I would want to hold on to this pain." And I know that that is what her conscious mind believed. However, when I asked her *subconscious* mind what was the reward it was receiving from being in pain all day, every day?

"My kids and grandkids won't come and visit me every weekend if I'm healthy," Alice said.

Do you see how massive this subconscious perceived reward is? If the belief is that by being healthy Alice would be all alone and never get to see her grandkids, why would Alice's subconscious ever allow her to become healthy?

I've seen this same pattern in countless clients.

How does one transform a belief this powerful that has been running the show automatically in the background for years? In Alice's case, the reward of releasing the pain has to be **greater** than getting to see her grandkids every week. That's a tall order! For example, letting the subconscious know that Alice wants to garden isn't going to cut it. It's not a big enough reward when compared with the prospect of loneliness. We had to make it crystal clear to Alice's subconscious that, yes, rather than seeing her grandkids every weekend, if she were healthy and comfortable (not in pain), it might be cut down to once a month. But without pain, she would **live longer** and get to spend more time with her grandkids **overall!**[52] She would increase her chances of getting to

52 Kristin Hayes, "Why Living in Pain Will Eventually Kill You," VeryWell Health, May 28, 2019, www.verywellhealth.com/why-living-in-pain-will -eventually-kill-you-3972227.

see those kiddos graduate high school, and get married, and even have babies themselves.

This point tipped the scales for Alice, and after a handful of hypnotherapy sessions, her pain went from an average of eight out of ten to an average of two out of ten.

Alice's experience illustrates that your subconscious has been clinging on to a reward that it believes is better than the reward you'll receive when you lose weight. **That** is one of the biggest reasons for why the weight has stayed put in the past despite all your efforts. That belief has to change.

Sugar: The Ultimate "Reward"

From our earliest memories, sugar is associated with all things positive: birthday cakes, a lollipop when you're a good little kid, ice cream when you come home with all A's on your report card, treats to help you stay quiet when your parents need a break. All this sugar releases dopamine into the brain.

With all this conditioning paired with dopamine being released, one's subconscious mind has *no* idea that sugar could be anything other than good for it. But, of course, we know that's not true. Sugar is not our friend. According to an article by NPR,

> The key player in the reward system of our brain—where we get that feeling of pleasure—is dopamine . . . Guess what happens when we eat sugar? Yes, those dopamine levels also surge . . . too much sugar too often can steer the brain into

overdrive... And that kickstarts a series of "unfortunate events"—loss of control, cravings and increased tolerance to sugar. All of those effects can be physically and psychologically taxing over time, leading to weight gain and dependence.[53]

The takeaway is pretty clear: if you're sensitive to sugar and inclined to indulge in a super-sugary treat, do it rarely and cautiously. Otherwise, there's a pretty good chance that your brain is going to start demanding sugar loudly and often. And you're better off without that extra voice in your head.

We all know the damaging effects of too much sugar consumption include weight gain,[54] energy

53 Eliza Barclay, "Why Sugar Makes Us Feel So Good," NPR, January 16, 2014, www.npr.org/sections/thesalt/2014/01/15/262741403/why-sugar-makes-us-feel -so-good.
54 V. S. Malik et al., "Sugar-Sweetened Beverages and Weight Gain in Children and Adults: A Systematic Review and Meta-analysis," *American Journal of Clinical Nutrition* 98, no. 4 (2013): 1084–1102, www.ncbi.nlm.nih.gov/ pubmed/23966427.

loss,[55] acceleration of cognitive decline,[56] acne,[57] type 2 diabetes,[58] and much more.[59]

This week's section in the bonus resources has an additional hypnosis recording that will help you navigate the slippery slope of sugar addiction. Robert, a long-time Grace Spacer, discovered from listening to this recording that he didn't have sugar *addiction* and that he simply needed to break down a bad habit of getting ice cream while walking home a few nights per week. Alice, on the other hand, was surprised to discover from the session that she felt controlled by sugar and that she needed to let go of it completely in order to feel free. She's since thrown away all sugar in the house. (Visit www.CloseYourEyesLoseWeight.com to listen and determine where you are on the scale.)

55 Donna Sprujit-Metz et al., "A High Sugar, Low Fiber Meal Leads to Higher Leptin and Physical Activity Levels in Overweight Latina Females as Opposed to a Low Sugar, High Fiber Meal," *Journal of the American Dietetic Association* 109, no. 6 (2009): 1058–63, www.ncbi.nlm.nih.gov/pmc/articles/PMC2768570/.
56 Paul K. Crane et al., "Glucose Levels and Risk of Dementia," *New England Journal of Medicine* 369, no. 19 (2013): 1863–64, www.nejm.org/doi/10.1056/NEJMc1311765.
57 Alicja Kucharska et al., "Significance of Diet in Treated and Untreated Acne Vulgaris," *Advances in Dermatology and Allergology* 33, no. 2 (2016): 81–86, www.ncbi.nlm.nih.gov/pmc/articles/PMC4884775/.
58 Sanjay Basu et al., "The Relationship of Sugar to Population-Level Diabetes Prevalence: An Econometric Analysis of Repeated Cross-Sectional Data," *PLoS One* 8, no. 2 (2013): e57873, www.ncbi.nlm.nih.gov/pmc/articles/PMC3584048/.
59 Jillian Kubala, "11 Reasons Why Too Much Sugar Is Bad for You," Healthline, June 3, 2018, www.healthline.com/nutrition/too-much-sugar.

I really like this passage from *Bright Line Eating* by Susan Pierce Thompson: "When *The Curious Case of Benjamin Button* came out, Brad Pitt and Cate Blanchett were on *Oprah*, and a fan who happened to be a chef . . . asked them what they most loved to eat. Both movie stars sat there, stumped. After several awkward moments, the best Cate Blanchett could muster was 'A bowl of rice is nice sometimes.' Brad Pitt chimed in with, 'Yeah, food's not really on my radar screen.'" Thompson uses this story to explain her method of understanding how strongly your brain reacts to the reward value of addictive foods. On Thompson's 1 to 10 susceptibility scale, Blanchett and Pitt would clearly score in the low susceptibility range (1 to 3). "If you're in the midrange (4 to 7), you may think of yourself as being somewhat challenged by food. If you're highly susceptible (8 to 10), you've probably struggled with your eating and/ or your weight for years, if not decades." Thompson declares, "Here's the simple truth. Plans based on moderation DO NOT work for people who are high on the Susceptibility Scale."[60]

I've found that my hypnotherapy clients who land on what Thompson deems as the mid-to-high susceptibility scale often require more conditioning than their lower-range counterparts when it comes to overcoming a feeling of deprivation or missing

---

60 Susan Pierce Thompson, *Bright Line Eating: The Science of Living Happy, Thin, and Free*, Carlsbad, CA: Hay House, Inc., 2017, 66-69.

out, but once that breakthrough happens, the feeling of freedom is absolutely paramount.

Wherever you land on the sugar-addiction scale or the susceptibility scale, letting the subconscious know that sugar (and carbs, dairy, etc.) are not *all good* is incredibly powerful in breaking the cycle of feeling powerless over foods that can be addictive.

It's common to hear extremes like, "Don't create negative associations with any foods; everything's good in moderation" (which is unhelpful to those who can't moderate), and "Anything other than organic broccoli is evil, treacherous poison" (which is unhelpful to those who have suffered from an eating disorder, including orthorexia—a medical condition in which the sufferer systematically and obsessively avoids specific foods in the belief that they are harmful). I will provide a wide range of suggestions that will help you reprogram your unique subconscious mind, based on your level of susceptibility, knowing that moderation does not work for everyone. It will be up to you to choose the affirmations that resonate most with your unique needs.

Sugar and Kids

Before we became parents, my husband and I made a lot of lofty declarations about all the sugar our kids would never, ever eat and the screens they would never, ever watch. How strong our convictions were! We hadn't yet sat through hours of screaming car rides or birthday parties where our little one would be the one toddler without frosting on their cheeks, crying that they want what the other kids are having, and realizing the carrot sticks we brought in the diaper bag weren't going to cut it this time. While we do limit sugar and screens a lot (they're not in the house), rather than avoiding them altogether and "demonizing" them to the point that we have sugar-and-phone-crazed teenagers rebelling against their parents' "antiquated ways," I took a page out of a dental hygienist's book. My dental hygienist friend told me that when her four kids were young, and she wanted them to behave, she would say, "If you're really, reallllly good, I'll let you brush your teeth when you get home!" When they pulled into the driveway of their home, four little rockets would shoot out of the back of the minivan, clambering over each other to be the first at the sink.

It's never easy knowing exactly what to do as a parent. It seems like whatever decision we make, there will be angry trolls on the internet vehemently disagreeing with that choice. But keep in mind that a big part of programming the subconscious mind in a helpful way is to program positive associations with helpful things. So if your kiddo does have sweets every now and again, do your best to make sure it isn't a big deal and that they aren't a reward. Here are some helpful alternatives that have worked for us: "If you're realllly good, I'll read you your favorite book when we get home!" "I have a special treat for you! It's apple slices with almond butter!" My son gets excited about this special treat of apple slices with almond butter because I get excited when I tell him about it. And if he does have a cupcake at a birthday party, he'll take a few bites and toss the rest. Sweets are not a big deal for him one way or another, which will make it much easier for him to make healthful decisions as an adult. It will be the same with your kids. And you're doing great already. Simply the fact that you're even considering the ways in which you talk about and present food to your kids, how it could be impacting their subconscious minds, is absolutely fantastic. Your little ones will thank you for it later.

· · · · · · · · · · · · · · · · ·

We can't stop addictive foods from being addictive. They either naturally are or have been engineered that way to elicit responses in the brain that say, "I need more!" What we do have control over is our ability to avoid addictive foods in the first place so we don't crave them later. We also have control over changing our idea of what an actual reward for good behavior is.

In what world would you reward yourself with something that makes you sick? Is diabetes a reward? Is heart failure a reward? Is high blood pressure or high cholesterol a reward? Of course not, but these are the effects of regularly eating unhelpful, addictive foods, including sugar.

The solution is to rewire our brains to see foods that lift us up, foods that give us energy, foods that make us feel amazing, as the

reward. In this week's hypnosis recording and self-hypnosis practice, that is exactly what you will do. The reward will no longer be what tastes good for one second and releases a fleeting dopamine hit. The reward will become nourishing your body with fuel that lifts you up. The reward will become eating foods that provide you with energy and long-term health. The reward will become spending time hiking when you're 85 or playing with your great-grandkids when you're 102 (like my nana is!).

The definition of poison is "a substance that is capable of causing the illness or death of a living organism when introduced or absorbed." It is not overdramatic to say that many "foods" were created in labs with the sole purpose of being addictive (certainly not with the purpose of having any nutritional value). These are poisonous. Lab-made foods might not be immediately lethal, but they're not contributing to a longer life span. Together, we will not let advertising or fake food trick us into "rewarding" ourselves with poison any longer. You deserve to consume life-*giving* foods.

In fact, you don't have to reward yourself with *food* at all! When your kids do a great job at school, reward them with stickers or a trip to the movies (bring your own helpful snacks). Reward yourself with a massage or get yourself a new journal. This week's hypnosis recording will also help you to get excited about rewards that have nothing to do with eating so food can go back to being simply **fuel** for your body. Take a nice, deep letting-go breath now and recognize that your body is a magnificent machine. You're a Porsche or a Maserati or a Tesla. You don't put crappy low-grade fuel into a Porsche. You decide now and forever to prioritize putting the highest quality fuel into your beautiful body.

Aversion Therapy

Aversion therapy is a type of hypnotherapy designed to make patients give up an undesirable habit by causing them to associate it with an unpleasant effect. This is especially effective when it comes to food. For example, imagine a table of sugary treats . . . crawling with hideous bugs. This does not create or manifest bugs in the real world, but it *does* create a powerful subconscious association with sugary treats being gross and undesirable. After a lifetime of conditioning and associations such as sugar equals birthday parties and rewards for good behavior, aversion therapy can be powerful in resetting the subconscious as to what is helpful or unhelpful to put into our bodies.

That said, for someone who has a history of orthorexia, this would potentially be triggering and not be anywhere near as helpful as focusing on the nourishing aspects of food. If a client of mine does **not** have a history of orthorexia or body dysmorphia, I have found that using aspects of aversion therapy can have powerful and positive results quickly. Know yourself, know what's right for you, and choose your hypno-affirmations accordingly. My team and I have labeled all bonus materials that use aversion therapy in case you prefer to skip it.

Homework

A. Practice self-hypnosis three times a day, every day this week (right before breakfast, lunch, and dinner). Turn to page 20 for a reminder of how to do self-hypnosis or head to www. CloseYourEyesLoseWeight.com to follow along with a tutorial video.

Week 7 Hypno-affirmations—Rewiring "Reward"

- I only consume foods that make my body feel loved for the long term.
- A true reward makes me feel great for the long term.
- A true reward supports my health for the long term.
- A punishment is something that hurts. Unhelpful foods are a punishment.
- I reward myself with healthy, nourishing foods.
- I am worthy and deserving of rewarding myself with _____ [insert helpful activity that is not eating].

B. Listen to the "Week 7—Rewiring Reward" hypnosis recording every day for the next week here: www. CloseYourEyesLoseWeight.com.

C. Use your journal pages daily to stay motivated, log your progress, and determine which pick-me-up hypno-affirmations you'll benefit from most.

Feels good, doesn't it? Choosing long-term joy and satisfaction over one-off dopamine hits that punish your body? I am so proud of you. Let's keep it going. In the pages ahead, I'll teach you how to avoid triggers that can lead to relapse, plus how to make helpful choices when facing temptation.

WEEK 7 LOG

TRACK YOUR PROGRESS

TODAY

Weight	Measurements		How Do You Feel in Your Clothes?	What's Your Energy Level?
	Neck:	Waist:		
	Chest:	Hips:	1 2 3 4 5	1 2 3 4 5
	(L) Arm	(L) Thigh:		
	(R) Arm	(R) Thigh:		

Write down any negative thoughts, immediately cross them out, and replace them with a positive thought.

CANCEL-CANCEL BOX

· ·
[PRO TIP] Stay neutral. Get curious!
· ·

How Will You Conjure Up Additional Energy When Needed?

10 jumping jacks ___   Shout hypno-affirmations ___   Other ___

Water

8oz of water before breakfast ___   8oz of water before lunch ___   8oz of water before dinner ___

This Morning's Self-Hypnosis | Round 1: Week 7—Rewiring "Reward"

Time you start: _____   Starting Stress Level (0–10): _____   Ending Stress Level (0–10): _____

This Afternoon's Self-Hypnosis | Round 2: Week 7—Rewiring "Reward"

Time you start: _____   Starting Stress Level (0–10): _____   Ending Stress Level (0–10): _____

This Evening's Self-Hypnosis | Round 3: Week 7—Rewiring "Reward"

Time you start: _____   Starting Stress Level (0–10): _____   Ending Stress Level (0–10): _____

Listen to this week's assigned hypnotherapy recording (found at www.CloseYourEyesLoseWeight.com): ☐

Tomorrow's Meal Planning

Breakfast	Snack	Lunch	Snack	Dinner

Check here when tomorrow's meals have been made or ordered: ☐

Visit www.CloseYourEyesLoseWeight.com and share your wins with our community: ☐

WEEK 7 LOG

TRACK YOUR PROGRESS

TODAY

Weight	Measurements		How Do You Feel in Your Clothes?	What's Your Energy Level?
	Neck:	Waist:		
	Chest:	Hips:	1 2 3 4 5	1 2 3 4 5
	(L) Arm	(L) Thigh:		
	(R) Arm	(R) Thigh:		

Write down any negative thoughts, immediately cross them out, and replace them with a positive thought.

CANCEL-CANCEL BOX

[PRO TIP] Stay neutral. Get curious!

How Will You Conjure Up Additional Energy When Needed?

10 jumping jacks ___   Shout hypno-affirmations ___   Other ___

Water

8oz of water before breakfast ___   8oz of water before lunch ___   8oz of water before dinner ___

This Morning's Self-Hypnosis | Round 1: Week 7—Rewiring "Reward"

Time you start: _____   Starting Stress Level (0–10): _____   Ending Stress Level (0–10): _____

This Afternoon's Self-Hypnosis | Round 2: Week 7—Rewiring "Reward"

Time you start: _____   Starting Stress Level (0–10): _____   Ending Stress Level (0–10): _____

This Evening's Self-Hypnosis | Round 3: Week 7—Rewiring "Reward"

Time you start: _____   Starting Stress Level (0–10): _____   Ending Stress Level (0–10): _____

Listen to this week's assigned hypnotherapy recording (found at www.CloseYourEyesLoseWeight.com): ☐

Tomorrow's Meal Planning

Breakfast	Snack	Lunch	Snack	Dinner

Check here when tomorrow's meals have been made or ordered: ☐

Visit www.CloseYourEyesLoseWeight.com and share your wins with our community: ☐

WEEK 7 LOG

TRACK YOUR PROGRESS

TODAY

Weight	Measurements		How Do You Feel in Your Clothes?	What's Your Energy Level?
	Neck:	Waist:		
	Chest:	Hips:	1 2 3 4 5	1 2 3 4 5
	(L) Arm	(L) Thigh:		
	(R) Arm	(R) Thigh:		

Write down any negative thoughts, immediately cross them out, and replace them with a positive thought.

CANCEL-CANCEL BOX

[PRO TIP] Stay neutral. Get curious!

How Will You Conjure Up Additional Energy When Needed?

10 jumping jacks ___   Shout hypno-affirmations ___   Other ___

Water

8oz of water before breakfast ___   8oz of water before lunch ___   8oz of water before dinner ___

This Morning's Self-Hypnosis | Round 1: Week 7—Rewiring "Reward"

Time you start: _____   Starting Stress Level (0–10): _____   Ending Stress Level (0–10): _____

This Afternoon's Self-Hypnosis | Round 2: Week 7—Rewiring "Reward"

Time you start: _____   Starting Stress Level (0–10): _____   Ending Stress Level (0–10): _____

This Evening's Self-Hypnosis | Round 3: Week 7—Rewiring "Reward"

Time you start: _____   Starting Stress Level (0–10): _____   Ending Stress Level (0–10): _____

Listen to this week's assigned hypnotherapy recording (found at www.CloseYourEyesLoseWeight.com): ☐

Tomorrow's Meal Planning

Breakfast	Snack	Lunch	Snack	Dinner

Check here when tomorrow's meals have been made or ordered: ☐

Visit www.CloseYourEyesLoseWeight.com and share your wins with our community: ☐

WEEK 7 LOG

DATE: __ / __ / __

TRACK YOUR PROGRESS

TODAY	Weight	Measurements		How Do You Feel in Your Clothes?	What's Your Energy Level?
		Neck:	Waist:		
		Chest:	Hips:	1 2 3 4 5	1 2 3 4 5
		(L) Arm	(L) Thigh:		
		(R) Arm	(R) Thigh:		

Write down any negative thoughts, immediately cross them out, and replace them with a positive thought.

CANCEL-CANCEL BOX

[PRO TIP] Stay neutral. Get curious!

How Will You Conjure Up Additional Energy When Needed?

10 jumping jacks ___   Shout hypno-affirmations ___   Other ___

Water

8oz of water before breakfast ___   8oz of water before lunch ___   8oz of water before dinner ___

This Morning's Self-Hypnosis | Round 1: Week 7—Rewiring "Reward"

Time you start: _____   Starting Stress Level (0–10): _____   Ending Stress Level (0–10): _____

This Afternoon's Self-Hypnosis | Round 2: Week 7—Rewiring "Reward"

Time you start: _____   Starting Stress Level (0–10): _____   Ending Stress Level (0–10): _____

This Evening's Self-Hypnosis | Round 3: Week 7—Rewiring "Reward"

Time you start: _____   Starting Stress Level (0–10): _____   Ending Stress Level (0–10): _____

Listen to this week's assigned hypnotherapy recording (found at www.CloseYourEyesLoseWeight.com): ☐

Tomorrow's Meal Planning

Breakfast	Snack	Lunch	Snack	Dinner

Check here when tomorrow's meals have been made or ordered: ☐

Visit www.CloseYourEyesLoseWeight.com and share your wins with our community: ☐

TRACK YOUR PROGRESS

TODAY

Weight	Measurements	How Do You Feel in Your Clothes?	What's Your Energy Level?
	Neck: Waist:		
	Chest: Hips:	1 2 3 4 5	1 2 3 4 5
	(L) Arm (L) Thigh:		
	(R) Arm (R) Thigh:		

Write down any negative thoughts, immediately cross them out, and replace them with a positive thought.

CANCEL-CANCEL BOX

[PRO TIP] Stay neutral. Get curious!

How Will You Conjure Up Additional Energy When Needed?

10 jumping jacks ___   Shout hypno-affirmations ___   Other ___

Water

8oz of water before breakfast ___   8oz of water before lunch ___   8oz of water before dinner ___

This Morning's Self-Hypnosis | Round 1: Week 7–Rewiring "Reward"

Time you start: _____   Starting Stress Level (0–10): _____   Ending Stress Level (0–10): _____

This Afternoon's Self-Hypnosis | Round 2: Week 7–Rewiring "Reward"

Time you start: _____   Starting Stress Level (0–10): _____   Ending Stress Level (0–10): _____

This Evening's Self-Hypnosis | Round 3: Week 7–Rewiring "Reward"

Time you start: _____   Starting Stress Level (0–10): _____   Ending Stress Level (0–10): _____

Listen to this week's assigned hypnotherapy recording (found at www.CloseYourEyesLoseWeight.com): ☐

Tomorrow's Meal Planning

Breakfast	Snack	Lunch	Snack	Dinner

Check here when tomorrow's meals have been made or ordered: ☐

Visit www.CloseYourEyesLoseWeight.com and share your wins with our community: ☐

WEEK 7 LOG

TRACK YOUR PROGRESS

TODAY

Weight	Measurements		How Do You Feel in Your Clothes?	What's Your Energy Level?
	Neck:	Waist:		
	Chest:	Hips:	1 2 3 4 5	1 2 3 4 5
	(L) Arm	(L) Thigh:		
	(R) Arm	(R) Thigh:		

Write down any negative thoughts, immediately cross them out, and replace them with a positive thought.

CANCEL-CANCEL BOX

. . . .

[PRO TIP] Stay neutral. Get curious!

. . . .

How Will You Conjure Up Additional Energy When Needed?

10 jumping jacks ___   Shout hypno-affirmations ___   Other ___

Water

8oz of water before breakfast ___   8oz of water before lunch ___   8oz of water before dinner ___

This Morning's Self-Hypnosis | Round 1: Week 7—Rewiring "Reward"

Time you start: _____   Starting Stress Level (0–10): _____   Ending Stress Level (0–10): _____

This Afternoon's Self-Hypnosis | Round 2: Week 7—Rewiring "Reward"

Time you start: _____   Starting Stress Level (0–10): _____   Ending Stress Level (0–10): _____

This Evening's Self-Hypnosis | Round 3: Week 7—Rewiring "Reward"

Time you start: _____   Starting Stress Level (0–10): _____   Ending Stress Level (0–10): _____

Listen to this week's assigned hypnotherapy recording (found at www.CloseYourEyesLoseWeight.com): ☐

Tomorrow's Meal Planning

Breakfast	Snack	Lunch	Snack	Dinner

Check here when tomorrow's meals have been made or ordered: ☐

Visit www.CloseYourEyesLoseWeight.com and share your wins with our community: ☐

TRACK YOUR PROGRESS

TODAY

Weight	Measurements	How Do You Feel in Your Clothes?	What's Your Energy Level?
	Neck: Waist:		
	Chest: Hips:		
	(L) Arm (L) Thigh:	1 2 3 4 5	1 2 3 4 5
	(R) Arm (R) Thigh:		

Write down any negative thoughts, immediately cross them out, and replace them with a positive thought.

CANCEL-CANCEL BOX

[PRO TIP] Stay neutral. Get curious!

How Will You Conjure Up Additional Energy When Needed?

10 jumping jacks ___   Shout hypno-affirmations ___   Other ___

Water

8oz of water before breakfast ___   8oz of water before lunch ___   8oz of water before dinner ___

This Morning's Self-Hypnosis | Round 1: Week 7—Rewiring "Reward"

Time you start: _____   Starting Stress Level (0–10): _____   Ending Stress Level (0–10): _____

This Afternoon's Self-Hypnosis | Round 2: Week 7—Rewiring "Reward"

Time you start: _____   Starting Stress Level (0–10): _____   Ending Stress Level (0–10): _____

This Evening's Self-Hypnosis | Round 3: Week 7—Rewiring "Reward"

Time you start: _____   Starting Stress Level (0–10): _____   Ending Stress Level (0–10): _____

Listen to this week's assigned hypnotherapy recording (found at www.CloseYourEyesLoseWeight.com): ☐

Tomorrow's Meal Planning

Breakfast	Snack	Lunch	Snack	Dinner

Check here when tomorrow's meals have been made or ordered: ☐

Visit www.CloseYourEyesLoseWeight.com and share your wins with our community: ☐

CHAPTER 11

. . . .

Week 8–
The People and Places
That Trigger You

When someone is getting sober, they identify the people and places that trigger the desire to use their drug of choice. It is powerful to model this as you rewire your brain to lose weight and love the body you have. The Starbucks drive-through on the way home? Your great-aunt's house? Your favorite ice cream place down the shore? When these people and places are consciously avoided, you will increase your likelihood of success. This is only until your conditioned neural pathways are strong enough to go there with your **new mindset** and habits firmly in place.

How do you find out what people and places trigger you to "use"? You could journal, tracking what you eat when you go to certain places or spend time with certain people. Those are great ideas, but they can take a long time. What's much faster? This week's hypnosis recording! You will be guided into a deeply relaxed state and then will be asked what and who your biggest triggers are. Once this is clear to you, the hypnosis session will guide you to make a plan of action as to how you can avoid these triggering people and places until your new subconscious beliefs and habits have become your new normal.

And the good news is, it won't take long! Yes, at first it can feel lonely, as if there is no one in the world who isn't a trigger. A common subconscious fear is, "If I just eat intuitively and chew, chew, chew, all family and friends will abandon me. No one will ever invite me to anything. They'll think I'm a snob or a weirdo." When your life is filled with heaping plates of carbs, cheese, sweets, salts, and everyone you spend time with also eats that way, it can be scary to imagine a life that's different. But only *before* hypnosis. That's because your brain does not yet have a frame of reference to imagine a different kind of life.

Once you commit to a new lifestyle, you will find out about the millions of people who already live that way. Healthy people who love what you love and think how you think can show you the way.

And one day, you can be that person for your family and friends. You can't turn others into what you want them to be, but you can show up and be a beacon of hope, an example of what's possible, a healthier way. When and if they're ready, they'll come to you for support. And when they do, I hope you'll hand them a copy of this book and say, "Come on, I'll take you to lunch where we can sit and chew together."

When You Can't Avoid the Trigger

What happens when you can't get out of visiting your great-aunt Mary's house, which you know will be filled to the brim with family favorites, all of which are not on your intuitive-eating list? Or the next coworker's birthday party with cake and brownies? Do you sit and sulk, feeling deprived? Do you have a bite? Do you say "ah screw it" and dig in? Do you happily abstain and eat the helpful snacks you brought with you? To be honest, your answer will depend on how much subconscious conditioning you've done *before* you arrive at the triggering locale.

So what if you do eat some unhelpful foods? Are you supposed to beat yourself up and feel negative and guilty so you "won't do it again"? Has beating yourself up *ever* stopped you from making that same unhelpful decision again, in the long term? I've never seen it work in even one of my over five thousand clients. Beating yourself up makes you feel bad. When you feel bad, what do you crave? Dopamine! When you crave dopamine, what do you do? Eat unhelpful things! How does that make you feel? Terrible! So, no, if you end up with a triggering person in a triggering place and you eat something unhelpful, here are the ways you get back on track ASAP; beating yourself up **isn't** one of them.

Watch out for the voice that says, "Well, I had a bite of brownie, so today's ruined. I'll start over tomorrow. In that case, I might as well have a huge scoop of the vodka penne, and these Swedish meatballs, and some of each kind of cheese, and at least a few bites of the three different pies she baked." That voice is digging the trench deeper. Just because you had a bite of brownie does *not* mean today is "ruined" and that you'll "start again tomorrow." You did not ruin everything, you still have all your faculties and total control over what you're going to do next.

My role is not to tell you "just have a bite of brownie. Enjoy it! It's all good. Life is for enjoyment." That's what advertisers tell you all day long. Life is a compilation of the choices you make over and over again. I'm here to help you make **new** choices, not give you a hall pass for old choices. At the same time, my role is not to tell you a bite of a brownie is morally reprehensible and now you must do penance! There is no value judgment here; it's about what is more helpful, less helpful, or what is unhelpful. My role is to help you reprogram your subconscious mind so you can lose weight and feel great. Given those parameters, here's what you do if you're faced with this situation:

1. "Cancel, cancel!" that voice of Resistance in your head that's saying you "ruined" today. It's telling you that so you'll eat with abandon for the rest of the day, and that will strengthen old neural pathways that you don't want to strengthen. "Cancel, cancel!" it and replace it with "I am safe, I am calm. Food is fuel. I only put the highest quality fuel into my miraculous body," then make sure your next choice of food is more helpful toward your goals.

2. Use the foundations you learned in chapter four, no matter what you're eating! Drink a glass of water before the bite of brownie. Chew that bite until only liquid remains. Whatever you're eating, make sure you stop when you're 90 percent satisfied. This applies to all foods, and it stops you from overeating anything, regardless of which category it comes from (unhelpful or helpful).

3. Use some aversion therapy while chewing and think about how unhealthy what you're eating is. If you affirm "Mmm, this is so good," you'll be triggering all those old habits you've worked so diligently to transform. It's not so good! No matter what it tastes like and no matter what dopamine it's releasing, if it's not good for you in the long term, don't you dare affirm "Mmm, this is so good" in

the now. "Cancel, cancel!" that and state the truth instead: "Yuck, there must be so many addictive synthetic ingredients in this. I'm so excited to make a more helpful choice next. I'm going to have a [insert helpful option] next."

Do you see how, even though you're eating the food, you're still programming your mind to think the way you *want* it to think? If aversion therapy doesn't feel good to you because of a history of orthorexia or other disordered eating, feel free to skip this step, but for those who haven't, this is a powerful way to weaken old, unhelpful neural pathways that we do not want strengthened.

I am so excited for you to listen to this week's hypnosis recording! Pretty soon your subconscious will have a powerful plan of action to avoid any triggering people and places. The more you avoid people and places where slip-ups are most likely to occur, especially in the beginning, the more you set yourself up for success. Realistically, sometimes these people, places, and things are unavoidable, so in those situations, put the fundamentals from chapter one to work and make sure you're always focused on what's more helpful with each and every choice.

Homework

A. Practice self-hypnosis three times a day, every day this week (right before breakfast, lunch, and dinner). Turn to page 20 for a reminder of how to do self-hypnosis or head to www.

CloseYourEyesLoseWeight.com to follow along with a tutorial video.

Week 8 Hypno-affirmations—Triggers: People and Places

- There are people I avoid so new, healthy habits have a chance to grow.
- There are places I avoid so new, healthy habits have a chance to grow.
- I seek out and spend time with people who eat helpful foods.
- I seek out people and places that help me succeed.
- Like someone who is getting sober, I avoid all triggers.
- I am kind to myself, come what may. Kindness is the fastest way to get back on track.

B. Listen to the "Week 8—Triggers: People & Places" hypnosis recording every day for the next week here: www.CloseYourEyesLoseWeight.com.

C. Use your journal pages daily to stay motivated, log your progress, and determine which pick-me-up hypno-affirmations you'll benefit from most.

• • • • • • • • • • • • • • • • • • • •

Congratulations! You now know who and what to avoid for the short term so those new neural pathways you're building have a chance to strengthen. You are now set up for success. If and when you happen to find yourself in an unavoidable triggering situation, you have a plan. You have the power. You have a choice. You're reprogramming your subconscious mind today so you are, in effect, making the right helpful choices in advance. Pat yourself on the back. In the next chapter, you're going to utilize the power of the law of attraction to manifest the body you desire, all while cherishing the body you have, today.

WEEK 8 LOG

TRACK YOUR PROGRESS

TODAY

Weight	Measurements	How Do You Feel in Your Clothes?	What's Your Energy Level?
	Neck: Waist:		
	Chest: Hips:	1 2 3 4 5	1 2 3 4 5
	(L) Arm (L) Thigh:		
	(R) Arm (R) Thigh:		

Write down any negative thoughts, immediately cross them out, and replace them with a positive thought.

CANCEL-CANCEL BOX

[PRO TIP] Stay neutral. Get curious!

How Will You Conjure Up Additional Energy When Needed?

10 jumping jacks ___   Shout hypno-affirmations ___   Other ___

Water

8oz of water before breakfast ___   8oz of water before lunch ___   8oz of water before dinner ___

This Morning's Self-Hypnosis | Round 1: Week 8—Triggers: People and Places

Time you start: _____   Starting Stress Level (0–10): _____   Ending Stress Level (0–10): _____

This Afternoon's Self-Hypnosis | Round 2: Week 8—Triggers: People and Places

Time you start: _____   Starting Stress Level (0–10): _____   Ending Stress Level (0–10): _____

This Evening's Self-Hypnosis | Round 3: Week 8—Triggers: People and Places

Time you start: _____   Starting Stress Level (0–10): _____   Ending Stress Level (0–10): _____

Listen to this week's assigned hypnotherapy recording (found at www.CloseYourEyesLoseWeight.com): ☐

Tomorrow's Meal Planning

Breakfast	Snack	Lunch	Snack	Dinner

Check here when tomorrow's meals have been made or ordered: ☐

Visit www.CloseYourEyesLoseWeight.com and share your wins with our community: ☐

WEEK 8 LOG

TRACK YOUR PROGRESS

TODAY

Weight	Measurements	How Do You Feel in Your Clothes?	What's Your Energy Level?
	Neck: Waist:		
	Chest: Hips:	1 2 3 4 5	1 2 3 4 5
	(L) Arm (L) Thigh:		
	(R) Arm (R) Thigh:		

Write down any negative thoughts, immediately cross them
out, and replace them with a positive thought.

CANCEL-CANCEL BOX

[PRO TIP] Stay neutral. Get curious!

How Will You Conjure Up Additional Energy When Needed?

10 jumping jacks ___   Shout hypno-affirmations ___   Other ___

Water

8oz of water before breakfast ___   8oz of water before lunch ___   8oz of water before dinner ___

This Morning's Self-Hypnosis | Round 1: Week 8–Triggers: People and Places

Time you start: _____   Starting Stress Level (0–10): _____   Ending Stress Level (0–10): _____

This Afternoon's Self-Hypnosis | Round 2: Week 8–Triggers: People and Places

Time you start: _____   Starting Stress Level (0–10): _____   Ending Stress Level (0–10): _____

This Evening's Self-Hypnosis | Round 3: Week 8–Triggers: People and Places

Time you start: _____   Starting Stress Level (0–10): _____   Ending Stress Level (0–10): _____

Listen to this week's assigned hypnotherapy recording (found at www.CloseYourEyesLoseWeight.com): ☐

Tomorrow's Meal Planning

Breakfast	Snack	Lunch	Snack	Dinner

Check here when tomorrow's meals have been made or ordered: ☐

Visit www.CloseYourEyesLoseWeight.com and share your wins with our community: ☐

WEEK 8 LOG

TRACK YOUR PROGRESS

TODAY

Weight	Measurements	How Do You Feel in Your Clothes?	What's Your Energy Level?
	Neck: _____ Waist: _____		
	Chest: _____ Hips: _____	1 2 3 4 5	1 2 3 4 5
	(L) Arm _____ (L) Thigh: _____		
	(R) Arm _____ (R) Thigh: _____		

Write down any negative thoughts, immediately cross them out, and replace them with a positive thought.

CANCEL-CANCEL BOX

[PRO TIP] Stay neutral. Get curious!

How Will You Conjure Up Additional Energy When Needed?

10 jumping jacks ___   Shout hypno-affirmations ___   Other ___

Water

8oz of water before breakfast ___   8oz of water before lunch ___   8oz of water before dinner ___

This Morning's Self-Hypnosis | Round 1: Week 8—Triggers: People and Places

Time you start: _____   Starting Stress Level (0–10): _____   Ending Stress Level (0–10): _____

This Afternoon's Self-Hypnosis | Round 2: Week 8—Triggers: People and Places

Time you start: _____   Starting Stress Level (0–10): _____   Ending Stress Level (0–10): _____

This Evening's Self-Hypnosis | Round 3: Week 8—Triggers: People and Places

Time you start: _____   Starting Stress Level (0–10): _____   Ending Stress Level (0–10): _____

Listen to this week's assigned hypnotherapy recording (found at www.CloseYourEyesLoseWeight.com): ☐

Tomorrow's Meal Planning

Breakfast	Snack	Lunch	Snack	Dinner

Check here when tomorrow's meals have been made or ordered: ☐

Visit www.CloseYourEyesLoseWeight.com and share your wins with our community: ☐

TRACK YOUR PROGRESS

TODAY

Weight	Measurements		How Do You Feel in Your Clothes?	What's Your Energy Level?
	Neck:	Waist:		
	Chest:	Hips:	1 2 3 4 5	1 2 3 4 5
	(L) Arm	(L) Thigh:		
	(R) Arm	(R) Thigh:		

Write down any negative thoughts, immediately cross them out, and replace them with a positive thought.

CANCEL-CANCEL BOX

[PRO TIP] Stay neutral. Get curious!

How Will You Conjure Up Additional Energy When Needed?

10 jumping jacks ___   Shout hypno-affirmations ___   Other ___

Water

8oz of water before breakfast ___   8oz of water before lunch ___   8oz of water before dinner ___

This Morning's Self-Hypnosis | Round 1: Week 8–Triggers: People and Places

Time you start: _____   Starting Stress Level (0–10): _____   Ending Stress Level (0–10): _____

This Afternoon's Self-Hypnosis | Round 2: Week 8–Triggers: People and Places

Time you start: _____   Starting Stress Level (0–10): _____   Ending Stress Level (0–10): _____

This Evening's Self-Hypnosis | Round 3: Week 8–Triggers: People and Places

Time you start: _____   Starting Stress Level (0–10): _____   Ending Stress Level (0–10): _____

Listen to this week's assigned hypnotherapy recording (found at www.CloseYourEyesLoseWeight.com): ☐

Tomorrow's Meal Planning

Breakfast	Snack	Lunch	Snack	Dinner

Check here when tomorrow's meals have been made or ordered: ☐

Visit www.CloseYourEyesLoseWeight.com and share your wins with our community: ☐

WEEK 8 LOG

TRACK YOUR PROGRESS

TODAY

Weight	Measurements		How Do You Feel in Your Clothes?	What's Your Energy Level?
	Neck:	Waist:		
	Chest:	Hips:		
	(L) Arm	(L) Thigh:	1 2 3 4 5	1 2 3 4 5
	(R) Arm	(R) Thigh:		

Write down any negative thoughts, immediately cross them out, and replace them with a positive thought.

CANCEL-CANCEL BOX

[PRO TIP] Stay neutral. Get curious!

How Will You Conjure Up Additional Energy When Needed?

10 jumping jacks ___   Shout hypno-affirmations ___   Other ___

Water

8oz of water before breakfast ___   8oz of water before lunch ___   8oz of water before dinner ___

This Morning's Self-Hypnosis | Round 1: Week 8—Triggers: People and Places

Time you start: _____   Starting Stress Level (0–10): _____   Ending Stress Level (0–10): _____

This Afternoon's Self-Hypnosis | Round 2: Week 8—Triggers: People and Places

Time you start: _____   Starting Stress Level (0–10): _____   Ending Stress Level (0–10): _____

This Evening's Self-Hypnosis | Round 3: Week 8—Triggers: People and Places

Time you start: _____   Starting Stress Level (0–10): _____   Ending Stress Level (0–10): _____

Listen to this week's assigned hypnotherapy recording (found at www.CloseYourEyesLoseWeight.com): ☐

Tomorrow's Meal Planning

Breakfast	Snack	Lunch	Snack	Dinner

Check here when tomorrow's meals have been made or ordered: ☐

Visit www.CloseYourEyesLoseWeight.com and share your wins with our community: ☐

WEEK 8 LOG

TRACK YOUR PROGRESS

TODAY

Weight	Measurements	How Do You Feel in Your Clothes?	What's Your Energy Level?
	Neck: Waist:		
	Chest: Hips:	1 2 3 4 5	1 2 3 4 5
	(L) Arm (L) Thigh:		
	(R) Arm (R) Thigh:		

Write down any negative thoughts, immediately cross them out, and replace them with a positive thought.

CANCEL-CANCEL BOX

[PRO TIP] Stay neutral. Get curious!

How Will You Conjure Up Additional Energy When Needed?

10 jumping jacks ___   Shout hypno-affirmations ___   Other ___

Water

8oz of water before breakfast ___   8oz of water before lunch ___   8oz of water before dinner ___

This Morning's Self-Hypnosis | Round 1: Week 8–Triggers: People and Places

Time you start: _____   Starting Stress Level (0–10): _____   Ending Stress Level (0–10): _____

This Afternoon's Self-Hypnosis | Round 2: Week 8–Triggers: People and Places

Time you start: _____   Starting Stress Level (0–10): _____   Ending Stress Level (0–10): _____

This Evening's Self-Hypnosis | Round 3: Week 8–Triggers: People and Places

Time you start: _____   Starting Stress Level (0–10): _____   Ending Stress Level (0–10): _____

Listen to this week's assigned hypnotherapy recording (found at www.CloseYourEyesLoseWeight.com): ☐

Tomorrow's Meal Planning

Breakfast	Snack	Lunch	Snack	Dinner

Check here when tomorrow's meals have been made or ordered: ☐

Visit www.CloseYourEyesLoseWeight.com and share your wins with our community: ☐

WEEK 8 LOG

TRACK YOUR PROGRESS

TODAY

Weight	Measurements	How Do You Feel in Your Clothes?	What's Your Energy Level?
	Neck: Waist:		
	Chest: Hips:	1 2 3 4 5	1 2 3 4 5
	(L) Arm (L) Thigh:		
	(R) Arm (R) Thigh:		

Write down any negative thoughts, immediately cross them out, and replace them with a positive thought.

CANCEL-CANCEL BOX

[PRO TIP] Stay neutral. Get curious!

How Will You Conjure Up Additional Energy When Needed?

10 jumping jacks ___   Shout hypno-affirmations ___   Other ___

Water

8oz of water before breakfast ___   8oz of water before lunch ___   8oz of water before dinner ___

This Morning's Self-Hypnosis | Round 1: Week 8—Triggers: People and Places

Time you start: _____   Starting Stress Level (0–10): _____   Ending Stress Level (0–10): _____

This Afternoon's Self-Hypnosis | Round 2: Week 8—Triggers: People and Places

Time you start: _____   Starting Stress Level (0–10): _____   Ending Stress Level (0–10): _____

This Evening's Self-Hypnosis | Round 3: Week 8—Triggers: People and Places

Time you start: _____   Starting Stress Level (0–10): _____   Ending Stress Level (0–10): _____

Listen to this week's assigned hypnotherapy recording (found at www.CloseYourEyesLoseWeight.com): ☐

Tomorrow's Meal Planning

Breakfast	Snack	Lunch	Snack	Dinner

Check here when tomorrow's meals have been made or ordered: ☐

Visit www.CloseYourEyesLoseWeight.com and share your wins with our community: ☐

PART IV

. . . .

Weeks 9–12

Progress Tracker

POUNDS LOST

Starting Weight _____

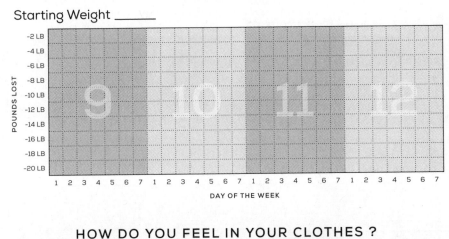

HOW DO YOU FEEL IN YOUR CLOTHES ?

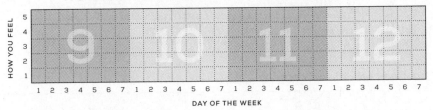

WHAT'S YOUR ENERGY LEVEL?

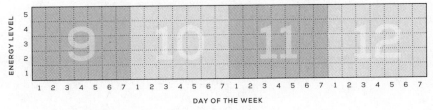

Starting Waist Measurement _____

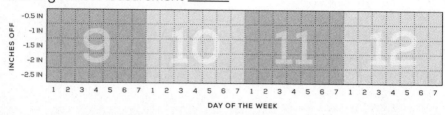

Starting Thigh (L) Measurement _____

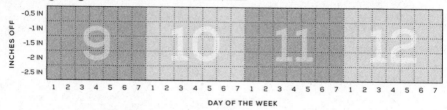

Starting Thigh (R) Measurement _____

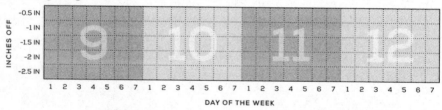

Starting Neck Measurement _____

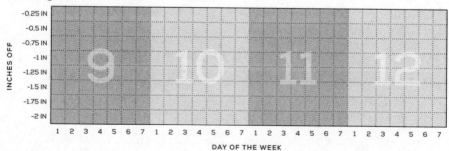

Starting Hip Measurement _____

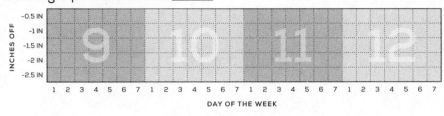

Starting Arm (L) Measurement _____

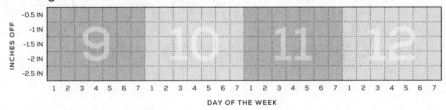

Starting Arm (R) Measurement _____

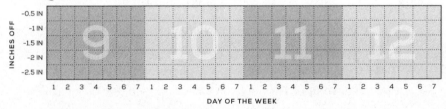

Starting Chest Measurement _____

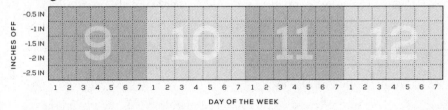

CHAPTER 12

· · · · · · · · · · · · · ·

Week 9–
Putting the Law of
Attraction to Work

You've completed two-thirds of your twelve-week journey, congratulations!

The law of attraction is the universal law that you attract into your life whatever you are focusing on. It was popularized by the book *The Secret*. If you focus on loving and appreciating the money you have, more money to love and appreciate is able to come your way. If you focus on *wanting* more money, opportunities to want money come your way (i.e., a need for money because a random bill arises without the funds to pay for it). In other words, stating what you really, really, really want is stating what you really, really, really don't have.

Sarah Prout is a world-renowned manifestation expert and the author of the international best seller *Dear Universe*.[61] In the course

---

61 For more information about Sarah, check out her website, https://sarahprout.com.

of researching this book, I had the opportunity to ask her a couple of questions: "What is it that most people don't understand about the law of attraction? And specifically, how can it help with something like weight loss when it seems to be mostly associated with things like manifesting a dream car?"

Sarah wrote back, "The traditional approach to manifesting and the law of attraction is the phrase 'thoughts become things'—but that's one piece of a much more complex puzzle. Your emotions are what construct the fabric of your reality—especially your physiology. When you feel good within your body *now*, with gratitude for your journey, and you work from there, then the Universe will respond with your intention." Isn't that amazing? Sarah had no idea that one of the pillars of this book is loving the body you *currently* have, and yet there it is, embedded in her message to you.

When cultivating the body you desire through self-love, you'll experience the fastest results by appreciating the body you have now, so you can continue to appreciate your body more and more in the future. If one were to focus on hating one's current body, via the law of attraction, in the future one will "attract" a body one can hate more and more.

With this in mind, think about the bodies you've compared yourself to your entire life. The ones you decided you wanted to look like. Who were you comparing yourself to? Who are you holding the vision of and telling the universe, "This is it! That is how beautiful, healthy humans are supposed to look!"?

If he or she isn't your height, within the same decade of your age, with your bone structure, and your hereditary makeup, you're likely setting yourself up for unnecessary pain and suffering.

If you are fifty-five years old, with DD cups and curly black hair, but Princess Kate is your standard of beauty and the person you want to emulate most, you would wake up every day and say to yourself, "I'm so ugly. I'm too old. I'm too fat. I look nothing like Princess Kate."

Or if you are 110 pounds with skin so fair you burn every time you step outside without sunscreen and have no curves to speak of, but Beyoncé is the standard of beauty you're holding yourself to, the cycle of feeling less-than will never stop.

What will those comparisons do? Via the law of attraction, you now know what kind of thoughts you will get more of.

More "ugly."

More "old."

More "fat."

More "Beyoncé and Princess Kate are the most beautiful of all." And implicit in that statement is "And since I'm nothing like them, I'll never be beautiful."

This is one of the reasons why representation matters. Why we need to see humans of every shape, size, and skin color in movies, on TV, on billboards, and in magazines . . . So we can begin to admire people we can anatomically emulate! It's fabulous to have a goal, but if I made my goal the measurement ratios of a voluptuous six-foot, buxom Victoria's Secret model, I would be sure to "fail."

Your healthy body, whatever size that means for you, is timeless. It is a classic. It is an unfading beauty.

In this week's self-hypnosis practice and hypnosis audio record-ing we'll use the power of the law of attraction to manifest the body you want, by falling in love with the miraculous body you have NOW.

Homework

A. Practice self-hypnosis three times a day, every day this week (right before breakfast, lunch, and dinner). Turn to page 20 for a reminder of how to do self-hypnosis or head to www. CloseYourEyesLoseWeight.com to follow along with a tutorial video.

Week 9 Hypno-affirmations—Law of Attraction

- I love my beautiful body exactly the way it is.
- My beautiful body and I love finding out what greatness we're capable of together.
- I love being _____
  [insert your current weight], and I love becoming _____ [insert your goal weight].
- I love [circle which ones you want to include] slim/ toned/fit/muscular people, and I wish them a long life filled with happiness. I am one of them.
- I love healthy people, and I wish them even more health and vitality. I am one of them.
- My body is a miracle, and I love every inch of it.

B. Listen to the "Week 9—Law of Attraction" hypnosis recording every day for the next week here: www. CloseYourEyesLoseWeight.com.

C. Use your journal pages daily to stay motivated, log your progress, and determine which pick-me-up hypno-affirmations you'll benefit from most.

D. Bonus Homework Assignment:
    Many people have difficulty visualizing their body in a way that is different from what it is now. If this describes your experience, I've got a bonus homework assignment for you.

This week's hypnosis session will help you to love the body you have and to visualize the best version of *your* body. Because that's what you're working so hard to cultivate and because that is what is naturally, anatomically possible for you. The best version of your body is not necessarily the same as the best version of Jennifer Lopez's body (because you are you, and Jennifer Lopez is Jennifer Lopez, and you are both not only perfect but also worthy of love and respect).

So here is your bonus homework assignment. Find an example of the "best," most vibrant, healthy version of *your* body that you would like to hold in your law of attraction visualization process so you can manifest it.

Magazines are still catching up slowly. (By the way, feel free to call out a publication that is lacking in diverse representation by reaching out to them on social media or via their customer support. Consumers have power, and if you decide to cancel a subscription owing to lack of representation, let the editors know it!) But you can do a quick image search or look on social media to find someone with a similar

- height (within one inch of your height);
- age (within ten years of your age); and
- similar prominent features (the things that don't change through weight loss).

This way when you look at this person as an indication of what's possible, it's also a believable

and achievable goal for you. This way you can
now use the law of attraction to your benefit as it
pertains to weight loss.

· · · · · · · · · · · · · · · ·

Utilizing the power of the law of attraction and your new frame of
reference for the body you desire to have, you are now able to clearly
visualize what you're manifesting while loving what you have.

The next chapter is for survivors of predatory behavior or sexual
abuse. There are many subconscious implications that these traumas
can have, and difficulty losing weight is one of them. While I wish
this chapter didn't have to exist, I have tremendous confidence that
healing the root of these issues will help set readers free. If chapter
ten's topic doesn't apply directly to you, you can skim it for helpful
information and then use this coming week to return to an area
that could benefit from an extra boost of conditioning. Return to
your data to see how you're tracking in each of our twelve core areas.
Spend this time on the area that needs the most support. If the topic
of chapter ten does apply to your direct life experience, this chapter
will likely be the one that has the greatest positive impact on your
life. I'm sending you love as we move forward together.

WEEK 9 LOG

TRACK YOUR PROGRESS

TODAY

Weight	Measurements		How Do You Feel in Your Clothes?	What's Your Energy Level?
	Neck:	Waist:		
	Chest:	Hips:	1 2 3 4 5	1 2 3 4 5
	(L) Arm	(L) Thigh:		
	(R) Arm	(R) Thigh:		

Write down any negative thoughts, immediately cross them out, and replace them with a positive thought.

CANCEL-CANCEL BOX

[PRO TIP] Stay neutral. Get curious!

How Will You Conjure Up Additional Energy When Needed?

10 jumping jacks ___   Shout hypno-affirmations ___   Other ___

Water

8oz of water before breakfast ___   8oz of water before lunch ___   8oz of water before dinner ___

This Morning's Self-Hypnosis | Round 1: Week 9—Law of Attraction

Time you start: _____   Starting Stress Level (0–10): _____   Ending Stress Level (0–10): _____

This Afternoon's Self-Hypnosis | Round 2: Week 9—Law of Attraction

Time you start: _____   Starting Stress Level (0–10): _____   Ending Stress Level (0–10): _____

This Evening's Self-Hypnosis | Round 3: Week 9—Law of Attraction

Time you start: _____   Starting Stress Level (0–10): _____   Ending Stress Level (0–10): _____

Listen to this week's assigned hypnotherapy recording (found at www.CloseYourEyesLoseWeight.com): ☐

Tomorrow's Meal Planning

Breakfast	Snack	Lunch	Snack	Dinner

Check here when tomorrow's meals have been made or ordered: ☐

Visit www.CloseYourEyesLoseWeight.com and share your wins with our community: ☐

WEEK 9 LOG

TRACK YOUR PROGRESS

TODAY

Weight	Measurements	How Do You Feel in Your Clothes?	What's Your Energy Level?
	Neck: Waist:		
	Chest: Hips:	1 2 3 4 5	1 2 3 4 5
	(L) Arm (L) Thigh:		
	(R) Arm (R) Thigh:		

Write down any negative thoughts, immediately cross them out, and replace them with a positive thought.

CANCEL-CANCEL BOX

[PRO TIP] Stay neutral. Get curious!

How Will You Conjure Up Additional Energy When Needed?

10 jumping jacks ___   Shout hypno-affirmations ___   Other ___

Water

8oz of water before breakfast ___   8oz of water before lunch ___   8oz of water before dinner ___

This Morning's Self-Hypnosis | Round 1: Week 9—Law of Attraction

Time you start: _____   Starting Stress Level (0–10): _____   Ending Stress Level (0–10): _____

This Afternoon's Self-Hypnosis | Round 2: Week 9—Law of Attraction

Time you start: _____   Starting Stress Level (0–10): _____   Ending Stress Level (0–10): _____

This Evening's Self-Hypnosis | Round 3: Week 9—Law of Attraction

Time you start: _____   Starting Stress Level (0–10): _____   Ending Stress Level (0–10): _____

Listen to this week's assigned hypnotherapy recording (found at www.CloseYourEyesLoseWeight.com): ☐

Tomorrow's Meal Planning

Breakfast	Snack	Lunch	Snack	Dinner

Check here when tomorrow's meals have been made or ordered: ☐

Visit www.CloseYourEyesLoseWeight.com and share your wins with our community: ☐

WEEK 9 LOG

TRACK YOUR PROGRESS

TODAY

Weight	Measurements	How Do You Feel in Your Clothes?	What's Your Energy Level?
	Neck: Waist:		
	Chest: Hips:		
	(L) Arm (L) Thigh:	1 2 3 4 5	1 2 3 4 5
	(R) Arm (R) Thigh:		

Write down any negative thoughts, immediately cross them out, and replace them with a positive thought.

CANCEL-CANCEL BOX

[PRO TIP] Stay neutral. Get curious!

How Will You Conjure Up Additional Energy When Needed?

10 jumping jacks ___   Shout hypno-affirmations ___   Other ___

Water

8oz of water before breakfast ___   8oz of water before lunch ___   8oz of water before dinner ___

This Morning's Self-Hypnosis | Round 1: Week 9—Law of Attraction

Time you start: _____   Starting Stress Level (0–10): _____   Ending Stress Level (0–10): _____

This Afternoon's Self-Hypnosis | Round 2: Week 9—Law of Attraction

Time you start: _____   Starting Stress Level (0–10): _____   Ending Stress Level (0–10): _____

This Evening's Self-Hypnosis | Round 3: Week 9—Law of Attraction

Time you start: _____   Starting Stress Level (0–10): _____   Ending Stress Level (0–10): _____

Listen to this week's assigned hypnotherapy recording (found at www.CloseYourEyesLoseWeight.com): ☐

Tomorrow's Meal Planning

Breakfast	Snack	Lunch	Snack	Dinner

Check here when tomorrow's meals have been made or ordered: ☐

Visit www.CloseYourEyesLoseWeight.com and share your wins with our community: ☐

TRACK YOUR PROGRESS

TODAY

Weight	Measurements	How Do You Feel in Your Clothes?	What's Your Energy Level?
	Neck: Waist:		
	Chest: Hips:		
	(L) Arm (L) Thigh:	1 2 3 4 5	1 2 3 4 5
	(R) Arm (R) Thigh:		

Write down any negative thoughts, immediately cross them out, and replace them with a positive thought.

CANCEL-CANCEL BOX

[PRO TIP] Stay neutral. Get curious!

How Will You Conjure Up Additional Energy When Needed?

10 jumping jacks ___   Shout hypno-affirmations ___   Other ___

Water

8oz of water before breakfast ___   8oz of water before lunch ___   8oz of water before dinner ___

This Morning's Self-Hypnosis | Round 1: Week 9—Law of Attraction

Time you start: _____   Starting Stress Level (0–10): _____   Ending Stress Level (0–10): _____

This Afternoon's Self-Hypnosis | Round 2: Week 9—Law of Attraction

Time you start: _____   Starting Stress Level (0–10): _____   Ending Stress Level (0–10): _____

This Evening's Self-Hypnosis | Round 3: Week 9—Law of Attraction

Time you start: _____   Starting Stress Level (0–10): _____   Ending Stress Level (0–10): _____

Listen to this week's assigned hypnotherapy recording (found at www.CloseYourEyesLoseWeight.com): ☐

Tomorrow's Meal Planning

Breakfast	Snack	Lunch	Snack	Dinner

Check here when tomorrow's meals have been made or ordered: ☐

Visit www.CloseYourEyesLoseWeight.com and share your wins with our community: ☐

WEEK 9 LOG

TRACK YOUR PROGRESS

TODAY

Weight	Measurements		How Do You Feel in Your Clothes?	What's Your Energy Level?
	Neck:	Waist:		
	Chest:	Hips:	1 2 3 4 5	1 2 3 4 5
	(L) Arm	(L) Thigh:		
	(R) Arm	(R) Thigh:		

Write down any negative thoughts, immediately cross them out, and replace them with a positive thought.

CANCEL-CANCEL BOX

[PRO TIP] Stay neutral. Get curious!

How Will You Conjure Up Additional Energy When Needed?

10 jumping jacks ___   Shout hypno-affirmations ___   Other ___

Water

8oz of water before breakfast ___   8oz of water before lunch ___   8oz of water before dinner ___

This Morning's Self-Hypnosis | Round 1: Week 9–Law of Attraction

Time you start: _____   Starting Stress Level (0–10): _____   Ending Stress Level (0–10): _____

This Afternoon's Self-Hypnosis | Round 2: Week 9–Law of Attraction

Time you start: _____   Starting Stress Level (0–10): _____   Ending Stress Level (0–10): _____

This Evening's Self-Hypnosis | Round 3: Week 9–Law of Attraction

Time you start: _____   Starting Stress Level (0–10): _____   Ending Stress Level (0–10): _____

Listen to this week's assigned hypnotherapy recording (found at www.CloseYourEyesLoseWeight.com): ☐

Tomorrow's Meal Planning

Breakfast	Snack	Lunch	Snack	Dinner

Check here when tomorrow's meals have been made or ordered: ☐

Visit www.CloseYourEyesLoseWeight.com and share your wins with our community: ☐

TRACK YOUR PROGRESS

TODAY

Weight	Measurements	How Do You Feel in Your Clothes?	What's Your Energy Level?
	Neck: Waist:		
	Chest: Hips:	1 2 3 4 5	1 2 3 4 5
	(L) Arm (L) Thigh:		
	(R) Arm (R) Thigh:		

Write down any negative thoughts, immediately cross them out, and replace them with a positive thought.

CANCEL-CANCEL BOX

[PRO TIP] Stay neutral. Get curious!

How Will You Conjure Up Additional Energy When Needed?

10 jumping jacks ___   Shout hypno-affirmations ___   Other ___

Water

8oz of water before breakfast ___   8oz of water before lunch ___   8oz of water before dinner ___

This Morning's Self-Hypnosis | Round 1: Week 9—Law of Attraction

Time you start: _____   Starting Stress Level (0–10): _____   Ending Stress Level (0–10): _____

This Afternoon's Self-Hypnosis | Round 2: Week 9—Law of Attraction

Time you start: _____   Starting Stress Level (0–10): _____   Ending Stress Level (0–10): _____

This Evening's Self-Hypnosis | Round 3: Week 9—Law of Attraction

Time you start: _____   Starting Stress Level (0–10): _____   Ending Stress Level (0–10): _____

Listen to this week's assigned hypnotherapy recording (found at www.CloseYourEyesLoseWeight.com): ☐

Tomorrow's Meal Planning

Breakfast	Snack	Lunch	Snack	Dinner

Check here when tomorrow's meals have been made or ordered: ☐

Visit www.CloseYourEyesLoseWeight.com and share your wins with our community: ☐

WEEK 9 LOG

TRACK YOUR PROGRESS

TODAY

Weight	Measurements		How Do You Feel in Your Clothes?	What's Your Energy Level?
	Neck:	Waist:		
	Chest:	Hips:		
	(L) Arm	(L) Thigh:	1 2 3 4 5	1 2 3 4 5
	(R) Arm	(R) Thigh:		

Write down any negative thoughts, immediately cross them out, and replace them with a positive thought.

CANCEL-CANCEL BOX

[PRO TIP] Stay neutral. Get curious!

How Will You Conjure Up Additional Energy When Needed?

10 jumping jacks __   Shout hypno-affirmations __   Other __

Water

8oz of water before breakfast __   8oz of water before lunch __   8oz of water before dinner __

This Morning's Self-Hypnosis | Round 1: Week 9—Law of Attraction

Time you start: _____   Starting Stress Level (0–10): _____   Ending Stress Level (0–10): _____

This Afternoon's Self-Hypnosis | Round 2: Week 9—Law of Attraction

Time you start: _____   Starting Stress Level (0–10): _____   Ending Stress Level (0–10): _____

This Evening's Self-Hypnosis | Round 3: Week 9—Law of Attraction

Time you start: _____   Starting Stress Level (0–10): _____   Ending Stress Level (0–10): _____

Listen to this week's assigned hypnotherapy recording (found at www.CloseYourEyesLoseWeight.com): ☐

Tomorrow's Meal Planning

Breakfast	Snack	Lunch	Snack	Dinner

Check here when tomorrow's meals have been made or ordered: ☐

Visit www.CloseYourEyesLoseWeight.com and share your wins with our community: ☐

CHAPTER 13

· · · · · · · · · · · · · · ·

Week 10–
How to Cope with
Unwanted Attention

This chapter is for survivors of sexual abuse or predatory behavior. Sexual abuse is one of the most consistent subconscious reasons I've seen amongst my clients to keep weight on and never let it go. The purpose of this chapter is to help you take your power back and live free from trauma, shame, and resentment. To help you live in a body that you have control over, a body that you are proud of. A body you love. A body that is your home and yours alone.

This is how weight loss, as strange as it might sound, can become a big, beautiful middle finger to an abuser who sought to rob you of your God-given peace and joy. Of your health. If this speaks to you, know that you no longer have to live in a cage built by someone else. You are worthy of being free. And it's time.

· · · · · · · · · · · · · ·

A common belief in the subconscious minds of many sexual abuse survivors is:

- being physically big in size = being invisible to society
- being invisible to society = being safe

I have seen this again and again with clients over the years. Research backs it up. A study by the American Academy of Pediatrics found that women who were sexually assaulted as children had nearly **double** the likelihood of becoming obese as an adult.[62]

Another common revelation for many weight loss hypnotherapy clients is that a subconscious part of them desires to keep the weight *on* so they might be less attractive to their partners. To lose weight would mean getting more attention and more advances from their own spouse, and their subconscious would do anything to avoid that. Another subconscious fear is that of the temptation to cheat on their spouse if they were to become more attractive.

There is a lot to unpack here. It's so much more than one chapter could ever cover because these subconscious beliefs are nuanced according to an individual's history and current circumstances. *If* this chapter applies to you, if you have experienced abuse in your past, or if you suspect you may be subconsciously keeping the weight on as a way of either avoiding sex with your partner, from a fear of straying, or to feel invisible (and therefore safe), this week's recording will be a welcome relief and a catalyst for tremendous healing.

---

62 Jennie G. Noll et al., "Obesity Risk for Female Victims of Childhood Sexual Abuse: A Prospective Study," *American Academy of Pediatrics* 120, no. 1 (2007): e61–e67, https://pediatrics.aappublications.org/content/120/1/e61.

. . . .

When the subconscious is blocking weight loss it is because it believes it is unsafe to receive attention. How do we heal this? You might think it would be to condition the subconscious mind with the belief that the world out there is safe. Unfortunately, we know that isn't always true, and our subconscious knows it too. There is no inherent value in my providing you with a hypno-affirmation like "You will never be assaulted," or "Catcalling is now illegal, and you will never feel unsafe walking home from work again." Still, you **must** decide you're not going to let the darkness in the world limit you. You are worthy of a bold, beautiful life, and yet it often takes tremendous courage to claim what is inherently yours.

For many of my New Yorker clients, flying post-9/11 was a terrifying prospect, and understandably so. A suggestion such as "it's safe to fly" or even "statistics say it's safer to fly than drive" would have fallen completely flat. The subconscious would simply reject it outright because there is truth to the fear that if something goes wrong with a flight, it's not the same as something going wrong when driving. We had to make the subconscious understand that the choice was between freedom or living a small life dictated by other people. The "reward" of flying again would have to become an act of defiance, an F-you to terrorism, a statement that they would never be allowed to win. This reframed flying from being something terrifying to being an act of courageous freedom. Sexual assault is terrorism. Allowing yourself to be healthy, sexy, to love your body, to live a bold, beautiful life is an act of defiance against those terrorists. By choosing your health, by choosing to love the body you have, you're setting yourself free from their terror.

Do you see how this kind of thinking helps you to reclaim your power?

You can't change anything with hypnosis but yourself. We can't stop the world from being a dangerous place with hypnosis (until, of course, everyone takes responsibility for their own mental health, healing, and upgrading of their individual subconscious programming).

But when we decide to commit ourselves to living a big, bold, beautiful life, to not let the darkness in the world dim our light, we can claim what's rightfully ours without subconscious fear. This week's hypnosis recording is here to help you heal from the past and reclaim your power in the present moment. It is here to help you feel safe and empowered in your body as it continues to lose weight. It is here to help you feel calm, confident, and safe even if you begin to receive more attention from strangers or your spouse or anyone else. It is here to help you reclaim your birthright as a sovereign being to live a beautiful, bold life and to look and feel however you damn well please while you do it. You deserve this. You always have, and you always will.

Homework

A. Practice self-hypnosis three times a day, every day this week (right before breakfast, lunch, and dinner). Turn to page 20 for a reminder of how to do self-hypnosis or head to www. CloseYourEyesLoseWeight.com to follow along with a tutorial video.

Week 10 Hypno-affirmations—Unwanted Attention

- I reclaim my power.
- I am safe; I am protected.
- It is safe for me to lose weight.
- I alone am the boss of my body.

- • I am perfect, whole, and complete.
- • I am worthy of a beautiful, bold, and healthy life.

B. Listen to the "Week 10–Unwanted Attention" hypnosis recording every day for the next week here: www.CloseYourEyesLoseWeight.com.

C. Use your journal pages daily to stay motivated, log your progress, and determine which pick-me-up hypno-affirmations you'll benefit from most.

．．．．．．．．．．．．．．．．

Your body is yours and yours alone. Your life is yours and yours alone. Your power is yours and yours alone. You are worthy of respect, of love. Now that you've taken this massive step forward towards breaking open any and all cages through the healing of past trauma, it's time to make sure your success can continue unimpeded. It's time to defeat the fear of success. We've come this far. Let's keep going. I believe in you.

WEEK 10 LOG

TRACK YOUR PROGRESS

TODAY

Weight	Measurements		How Do You Feel in Your Clothes?	What's Your Energy Level?
	Neck:	Waist:		
	Chest:	Hips:	1 2 3 4 5	1 2 3 4 5
	(L) Arm	(L) Thigh:		
	(R) Arm	(R) Thigh:		

Write down any negative thoughts, immediately cross them out, and replace them with a positive thought.

CANCEL-CANCEL BOX

[PRO TIP] Stay neutral. Get curious!

How Will You Conjure Up Additional Energy When Needed?

10 jumping jacks ___   Shout hypno-affirmations ___   Other ___

Water

8oz of water before breakfast ___   8oz of water before lunch ___   8oz of water before dinner ___

This Morning's Self-Hypnosis | Round 1: Week 10—Unwanted Attention

Time you start: _____   Starting Stress Level (0–10): _____   Ending Stress Level (0–10): _____

This Afternoon's Self-Hypnosis | Round 2: Week 10—Unwanted Attention

Time you start: _____   Starting Stress Level (0–10): _____   Ending Stress Level (0–10): _____

This Evening's Self-Hypnosis | Round 3: Week 10—Unwanted Attention

Time you start: _____   Starting Stress Level (0–10): _____   Ending Stress Level (0–10): _____

Listen to this week's assigned hypnotherapy recording (found at www.CloseYourEyesLoseWeight.com): ☐

Tomorrow's Meal Planning

Breakfast	Snack	Lunch	Snack	Dinner

Check here when tomorrow's meals have been made or ordered: ☐

Visit www.CloseYourEyesLoseWeight.com and share your wins with our community: ☐

WEEK 10 LOG

TRACK YOUR PROGRESS

TODAY

Weight	Measurements		How Do You Feel in Your Clothes?	What's Your Energy Level?
	Neck:	Waist:		
	Chest:	Hips:	1 2 3 4 5	1 2 3 4 5
	(L) Arm	(L) Thigh:		
	(R) Arm	(R) Thigh:		

Write down any negative thoughts, immediately cross them out, and replace them with a positive thought.

CANCEL-CANCEL BOX

[PRO TIP] Stay neutral. Get curious!

How Will You Conjure Up Additional Energy When Needed?

10 jumping jacks ___   Shout hypno-affirmations ___   Other ___

Water

8oz of water before breakfast ___   8oz of water before lunch ___   8oz of water before dinner ___

This Morning's Self-Hypnosis | Round 1: Week 10—Unwanted Attention

Time you start: _____   Starting Stress Level (0–10): _____   Ending Stress Level (0–10): _____

This Afternoon's Self-Hypnosis | Round 2: Week 10—Unwanted Attention

Time you start: _____   Starting Stress Level (0–10): _____   Ending Stress Level (0–10): _____

This Evening's Self-Hypnosis | Round 3: Week 10—Unwanted Attention

Time you start: _____   Starting Stress Level (0–10): _____   Ending Stress Level (0–10): _____

Listen to this week's assigned hypnotherapy recording (found at www.CloseYourEyesLoseWeight.com): ☐

Tomorrow's Meal Planning

Breakfast	Snack	Lunch	Snack	Dinner

Check here when tomorrow's meals have been made or ordered: ☐

Visit www.CloseYourEyesLoseWeight.com and share your wins with our community: ☐

TRACK YOUR PROGRESS

TODAY

Weight	Measurements	How Do You Feel in Your Clothes?	What's Your Energy Level?
	Neck: Waist:		
	Chest: Hips:	1 2 3 4 5	1 2 3 4 5
	(L) Arm (L) Thigh:		
	(R) Arm (R) Thigh:		

Write down any negative thoughts, immediately cross them out, and replace them with a positive thought.

CANCEL-CANCEL BOX

[PRO TIP] Stay neutral. Get curious!

How Will You Conjure Up Additional Energy When Needed?

10 jumping jacks ___   Shout hypno-affirmations ___   Other ___

Water

8oz of water before breakfast ___   8oz of water before lunch ___   8oz of water before dinner ___

This Morning's Self-Hypnosis | Round 1: Week 10–Unwanted Attention

Time you start: _____   Starting Stress Level (0–10): _____   Ending Stress Level (0–10): _____

This Afternoon's Self-Hypnosis | Round 2: Week 10–Unwanted Attention

Time you start: _____   Starting Stress Level (0–10): _____   Ending Stress Level (0–10): _____

This Evening's Self-Hypnosis | Round 3: Week 10–Unwanted Attention

Time you start: _____   Starting Stress Level (0–10): _____   Ending Stress Level (0–10): _____

Listen to this week's assigned hypnotherapy recording (found at www.CloseYourEyesLoseWeight.com): ☐

Tomorrow's Meal Planning

Breakfast	Snack	Lunch	Snack	Dinner

Check here when tomorrow's meals have been made or ordered: ☐

Visit www.CloseYourEyesLoseWeight.com and share your wins with our community: ☐

WEEK 10 LOG

TRACK YOUR PROGRESS

TODAY

Weight	Measurements	How Do You Feel in Your Clothes?	What's Your Energy Level?
	Neck: Waist:		
	Chest: Hips:	1 2 3 4 5	1 2 3 4 5
	(L) Arm (L) Thigh:		
	(R) Arm (R) Thigh:		

Write down any negative thoughts, immediately cross them out, and replace them with a positive thought.

CANCEL-CANCEL BOX

[PRO TIP] Stay neutral. Get curious!

How Will You Conjure Up Additional Energy When Needed?

10 jumping jacks ___   Shout hypno-affirmations ___   Other ___

Water

8oz of water before breakfast ___   8oz of water before lunch ___   8oz of water before dinner ___

This Morning's Self-Hypnosis | Round 1: Week 10—Unwanted Attention

Time you start: _____   Starting Stress Level (0–10): _____   Ending Stress Level (0–10): _____

This Afternoon's Self-Hypnosis | Round 2: Week 10—Unwanted Attention

Time you start: _____   Starting Stress Level (0–10): _____   Ending Stress Level (0–10): _____

This Evening's Self-Hypnosis | Round 3: Week 10—Unwanted Attention

Time you start: _____   Starting Stress Level (0–10): _____   Ending Stress Level (0–10): _____

Listen to this week's assigned hypnotherapy recording (found at www.CloseYourEyesLoseWeight.com): ☐

Tomorrow's Meal Planning

Breakfast	Snack	Lunch	Snack	Dinner

Check here when tomorrow's meals have been made or ordered: ☐

Visit www.CloseYourEyesLoseWeight.com and share your wins with our community: ☐

WEEK 10 LOG

TRACK YOUR PROGRESS

TODAY

Weight	Measurements	How Do You Feel in Your Clothes?	What's Your Energy Level?
	Neck: Waist:		
	Chest: Hips:	1 2 3 4 5	1 2 3 4 5
	(L) Arm (L) Thigh:		
	(R) Arm (R) Thigh:		

Write down any negative thoughts, immediately cross them out, and replace them with a positive thought.

CANCEL-CANCEL BOX

[PRO TIP] Stay neutral. Get curious!

How Will You Conjure Up Additional Energy When Needed?

10 jumping jacks ___   Shout hypno-affirmations ___   Other ___

Water

8oz of water before breakfast ___   8oz of water before lunch ___   8oz of water before dinner ___

This Morning's Self-Hypnosis | Round 1: Week 10—Unwanted Attention

Time you start: _____   Starting Stress Level (0–10): _____   Ending Stress Level (0–10): _____

This Afternoon's Self-Hypnosis | Round 2: Week 10—Unwanted Attention

Time you start: _____   Starting Stress Level (0–10): _____   Ending Stress Level (0–10): _____

This Evening's Self-Hypnosis | Round 3: Week 10—Unwanted Attention

Time you start: _____   Starting Stress Level (0–10): _____   Ending Stress Level (0–10): _____

Listen to this week's assigned hypnotherapy recording (found at www.CloseYourEyesLoseWeight.com): ☐

Tomorrow's Meal Planning

Breakfast	Snack	Lunch	Snack	Dinner

Check here when tomorrow's meals have been made or ordered: ☐

Visit www.CloseYourEyesLoseWeight.com and share your wins with our community: ☐

WEEK 10 LOG

TRACK YOUR PROGRESS

TODAY

Weight	Measurements		How Do You Feel in Your Clothes?	What's Your Energy Level?
	Neck:	Waist:		
	Chest:	Hips:	1 2 3 4 5	1 2 3 4 5
	(L) Arm	(L) Thigh:		
	(R) Arm	(R) Thigh:		

Write down any negative thoughts, immediately cross them out, and replace them with a positive thought.

CANCEL-CANCEL BOX

[PRO TIP] Stay neutral. Get curious!

How Will You Conjure Up Additional Energy When Needed?

10 jumping jacks ___   Shout hypno-affirmations ___   Other ___

Water

8oz of water before breakfast ___   8oz of water before lunch ___   8oz of water before dinner ___

This Morning's Self-Hypnosis | Round 1: Week 10—Unwanted Attention

Time you start: _____   Starting Stress Level (0–10): _____   Ending Stress Level (0–10): _____

This Afternoon's Self-Hypnosis | Round 2: Week 10—Unwanted Attention

Time you start: _____   Starting Stress Level (0–10): _____   Ending Stress Level (0–10): _____

This Evening's Self-Hypnosis | Round 3: Week 10—Unwanted Attention

Time you start: _____   Starting Stress Level (0–10): _____   Ending Stress Level (0–10): _____

Listen to this week's assigned hypnotherapy recording (found at www.CloseYourEyesLoseWeight.com): ☐

Tomorrow's Meal Planning

Breakfast	Snack	Lunch	Snack	Dinner

Check here when tomorrow's meals have been made or ordered: ☐

Visit www.CloseYourEyesLoseWeight.com and share your wins with our community: ☐

WEEK 10 LOG

TRACK YOUR PROGRESS

TODAY

Weight	Measurements	How Do You Feel in Your Clothes?	What's Your Energy Level?
	Neck: Waist:		
	Chest: Hips:	1 2 3 4 5	1 2 3 4 5
	(L) Arm (L) Thigh:		
	(R) Arm (R) Thigh:		

Write down any negative thoughts, immediately cross them out, and replace them with a positive thought.

CANCEL-CANCEL BOX

· ·

[PRO TIP] Stay neutral. Get curious!

· ·

How Will You Conjure Up Additional Energy When Needed?

10 jumping jacks ___   Shout hypno-affirmations ___   Other ___

Water

8oz of water before breakfast ___   8oz of water before lunch ___   8oz of water before dinner ___

This Morning's Self-Hypnosis | Round 1: Week 10—Unwanted Attention

Time you start: _____   Starting Stress Level (0–10): _____   Ending Stress Level (0–10): _____

This Afternoon's Self-Hypnosis | Round 2: Week 10—Unwanted Attention

Time you start: _____   Starting Stress Level (0–10): _____   Ending Stress Level (0–10): _____

This Evening's Self-Hypnosis | Round 3: Week 10—Unwanted Attention

Time you start: _____   Starting Stress Level (0–10): _____   Ending Stress Level (0–10): _____

Listen to this week's assigned hypnotherapy recording (found at www.CloseYourEyesLoseWeight.com): ☐

Tomorrow's Meal Planning

Breakfast	Snack	Lunch	Snack	Dinner

Check here when tomorrow's meals have been made or ordered: ☐

Visit www.CloseYourEyesLoseWeight.com and share your wins with our community: ☐

CHAPTER 14

· · · · · · · · · · · · · · · · · · ·

Week 11– Overcome the Fear of Success

> "I'm honestly doing this because I want to change my mindset permanently and make healthy choices every day." –Alesha C., Bronx, New York

At this point, since you've been listening to your weekly hypnosis recordings, and practicing your self-hypnosis three times per day, you're likely beginning to experience some incredible results. Congratulations—you deserve this!

And beware, *this* is the moment when Resistance loves to pop back up again.

What to watch out for:

"You did it! You're looking great. What could a piece of x, y, z possibly do to you now? You're on a roll. You 'deserve' to have x, y, z to 'congratulate' yourself."

THIS IS SELF-SABOTAGE. RUN IN THE OTHER DIRECTION!

There is no reason to ever celebrate or "congratulate" yourself with something that causes you harm in the long run. If these thoughts start to pop up, do ten jumping jacks or roll up on your toes ten times, reaching up to the ceiling with your fingertips. Drink a big glass of water and take a few deep, slow breaths before deciding on what helpful action you'd like to take next.

Ask yourself, "Will consuming x, y, z make me feel good in the long term? Will it support my health in the long term?" If the answer is no, you know what to do. If the answer is yes, go for it, and chew, chew, chew!

The subconscious wants you to believe that your weight loss journey is a race. It's a race it never wanted you to sign up for, but you did. And you're running it. You're losing weight. You're falling in love with your body. And now Resistance wants you to think you just ran through the yellow tape, your arms spread wide like wings, your face beaming as you tilt back your head and smile up at the sun. Resistance wants you to believe that the race is over now, that it's time to finally go back to sitting on the couch in loose sweats, bingeing on Netflix, and consuming unhelpful foods by the fistful.

I repeat, THIS IS SELF-SABOTAGE! *This* is where the weight loss–weight gain–weight loss–weight gain yo-yo often begins. But not for you! Not this time. You. Are. Not. Doing. That. Take out a hammer and smash that yo-yo to bits. This is the time to double down on your recordings and review the data you've been tracking in the journal section to see what areas will benefit from additional conditioning.

When losing weight stops being something you're "trying" to do, or something you "want" to do, and it becomes what you're *doing*, the subconscious is going to give another last-ditch effort to get things back to the way they used to be. Don't let it.

Your journey is not a race. It's not even a marathon; even the longest marathons end after a few days. This is your entire life. You have come so far, and yet you must continue. You are worthy of continuing. Return to your intake form on page 52 and remind yourself why this is so important to you. Resistance is the hump to get over. The times when you feel success and breakthroughs are some of the most vulnerable times. That's when you need to recognize self-sabotage for what it is and stop it in its tracks.

This week's hypnosis recording is nice and short. The purpose of it is to reset your subconscious mind to release Resistance and get back on track! Listen to it as a booster and then follow it up with the week's recording that your data indicates you'll benefit from the most.

Homework

A. Practice self-hypnosis three times a day, every day this week (right before breakfast, lunch, and dinner). Turn to page 20 for a reminder of how to do self-hypnosis or head to www. CloseYourEyesLoseWeight.com to follow along with a tutorial video.

Week 11 Hypno-affirmations—Keep Going, Beat Resistance

- It is safe for success to be my new normal.
- I am doing great and commit to keep going.

- I am proud of myself for continuing this beautiful journey.
- I am the same wonderful person, with an upgraded exterior.
- I am worthy of continuing.
- I cultivate energy, get motivated, stay vigilant, and beat Resistance!

B. Listen to the short "Keep Going, Overcome Resistance!" booster hypnosis recording (found at www.CloseYourEyesLoseWeight.com) right before returning to a week where you need the most amount of additional support and listening to that recording.
  It could look like this:
  Monday: "Keep Going!" Recording + Motivation Recording
  Tuesday: "Keep Going!" Recording + Foundations Recording
  Wednesday: "Keep Going!" Recording + Limiting Beliefs
  And so on and so forth for Thursday through Sunday
C. Use your journal pages daily to stay motivated, log your progress, and determine which pick-me-up hypno-affirmations you'll benefit from most.

I'm proud of you. I believe in you. You are worthy and deserving of doubling down on your efforts and experiencing a lifetime of choices that support the highest version, the highest expression of who you are.

Keep going!

True love is a journey. Self-love is no different. As you reach new milestones on your weight loss journey, celebrate them. Celebrate *you*. And release self-sabotaging beliefs and behaviors that masquerade as rewards. Success is its own reward. Your body deserves to be adored, to be cared for, to be loved. In week twelve, you'll come to appreciate everything about your body, even parts you probably never thought to thank before. Turn the page!

TRACK YOUR PROGRESS

TODAY

Weight	Measurements	How Do You Feel in Your Clothes?	What's Your Energy Level?
	Neck: Waist:		
	Chest: Hips:	1 2 3 4 5	1 2 3 4 5
	(L) Arm (L) Thigh:		
	(R) Arm (R) Thigh:		

Write down any negative thoughts, immediately cross them out, and replace them with a positive thought.

CANCEL-CANCEL BOX

[PRO TIP] Stay neutral. Get curious!

How Will You Conjure Up Additional Energy When Needed?

10 jumping jacks ___   Shout hypno-affirmations ___   Other ___

Water

8oz of water before breakfast ___   8oz of water before lunch ___   8oz of water before dinner ___

This Morning's Self-Hypnosis | Round 1: Week 11–Keep Going, Beat Resistance

Time you start: _____   Starting Stress Level (0–10): _____   Ending Stress Level (0–10): _____

This Afternoon's Self-Hypnosis | Round 2: Week 11–Keep Going, Beat Resistance

Time you start: _____   Starting Stress Level (0–10): _____   Ending Stress Level (0–10): _____

This Evening's Self-Hypnosis | Round 3: Week 11–Keep Going, Beat Resistance

Time you start: _____   Starting Stress Level (0–10): _____   Ending Stress Level (0–10): _____

Listen to this week's assigned hypnotherapy recording (found at www.CloseYourEyesLoseWeight.com): ☐

Tomorrow's Meal Planning

Breakfast	Snack	Lunch	Snack	Dinner

Check here when tomorrow's meals have been made or ordered: ☐

Visit www.CloseYourEyesLoseWeight.com and share your wins with our community: ☐

WEEK 11 LOG

TRACK YOUR PROGRESS

TODAY

Weight	Measurements	How Do You Feel in Your Clothes?	What's Your Energy Level?
	Neck: Waist:		
	Chest: Hips:	1 2 3 4 5	1 2 3 4 5
	(L) Arm (L) Thigh:		
	(R) Arm (R) Thigh:		

Write down any negative thoughts, immediately cross them out, and replace them with a positive thought.

CANCEL-CANCEL BOX

[PRO TIP] Stay neutral. Get curious!

How Will You Conjure Up Additional Energy When Needed?

10 jumping jacks __   Shout hypno-affirmations __   Other __

Water

8oz of water before breakfast __   8oz of water before lunch __   8oz of water before dinner __

This Morning's Self-Hypnosis | Round 1: Week 11—Keep Going, Beat Resistance

Time you start: _____   Starting Stress Level (0–10): _____   Ending Stress Level (0–10): _____

This Afternoon's Self-Hypnosis | Round 2: Week 11—Keep Going, Beat Resistance

Time you start: _____   Starting Stress Level (0–10): _____   Ending Stress Level (0–10): _____

This Evening's Self-Hypnosis | Round 3: Week 11—Keep Going, Beat Resistance

Time you start: _____   Starting Stress Level (0–10): _____   Ending Stress Level (0–10): _____

Listen to this week's assigned hypnotherapy recording (found at www.CloseYourEyesLoseWeight.com): ☐

Tomorrow's Meal Planning

Breakfast	Snack	Lunch	Snack	Dinner

Check here when tomorrow's meals have been made or ordered: ☐

Visit www.CloseYourEyesLoseWeight.com and share your wins with our community: ☐

WEEK 11 LOG

TRACK YOUR PROGRESS

TODAY

Weight	Measurements	How Do You Feel in Your Clothes?	What's Your Energy Level?
	Neck: Waist:		
	Chest: Hips:	1 2 3 4 5	1 2 3 4 5
	(L) Arm (L) Thigh:		
	(R) Arm (R) Thigh:		

Write down any negative thoughts, immediately cross them out, and replace them with a positive thought.

CANCEL-CANCEL BOX

[PRO TIP] Stay neutral. Get curious!

How Will You Conjure Up Additional Energy When Needed?

10 jumping jacks ___   Shout hypno-affirmations ___   Other ___

Water

8oz of water before breakfast ___   8oz of water before lunch ___   8oz of water before dinner ___

This Morning's Self-Hypnosis | Round 1: Week 11–Keep Going, Beat Resistance

Time you start: _____   Starting Stress Level (0–10): _____   Ending Stress Level (0–10): _____

This Afternoon's Self-Hypnosis | Round 2: Week 11–Keep Going, Beat Resistance

Time you start: _____   Starting Stress Level (0–10): _____   Ending Stress Level (0–10): _____

This Evening's Self-Hypnosis | Round 3: Week 11–Keep Going, Beat Resistance

Time you start: _____   Starting Stress Level (0–10): _____   Ending Stress Level (0–10): _____

Listen to this week's assigned hypnotherapy recording (found at www.CloseYourEyesLoseWeight.com): ☐

Tomorrow's Meal Planning

Breakfast	Snack	Lunch	Snack	Dinner

Check here when tomorrow's meals have been made or ordered: ☐

Visit www.CloseYourEyesLoseWeight.com and share your wins with our community: ☐

TRACK YOUR PROGRESS

TODAY

Weight	Measurements		How Do You Feel in Your Clothes?	What's Your Energy Level?
	Neck:	Waist:		
	Chest:	Hips:	1 2 3 4 5	1 2 3 4 5
	(L) Arm	(L) Thigh:		
	(R) Arm	(R) Thigh:		

Write down any negative thoughts, immediately cross them out, and replace them with a positive thought.

CANCEL-CANCEL BOX

[PRO TIP] Stay neutral. Get curious!

How Will You Conjure Up Additional Energy When Needed?

10 jumping jacks ___   Shout hypno-affirmations ___   Other ___

Water

8oz of water before breakfast ___   8oz of water before lunch ___   8oz of water before dinner ___

This Morning's Self-Hypnosis | Round 1: Week 11—Keep Going, Beat Resistance

Time you start: _____   Starting Stress Level (0–10): _____   Ending Stress Level (0–10): _____

This Afternoon's Self-Hypnosis | Round 2: Week 11—Keep Going, Beat Resistance

Time you start: _____   Starting Stress Level (0–10): _____   Ending Stress Level (0–10): _____

This Evening's Self-Hypnosis | Round 3: Week 11—Keep Going, Beat Resistance

Time you start: _____   Starting Stress Level (0–10): _____   Ending Stress Level (0–10): _____

Listen to this week's assigned hypnotherapy recording (found at www.CloseYourEyesLoseWeight.com): ☐

Tomorrow's Meal Planning

Breakfast	Snack	Lunch	Snack	Dinner

Check here when tomorrow's meals have been made or ordered: ☐

Visit www.CloseYourEyesLoseWeight.com and share your wins with our community: ☐

WEEK 11 LOG

TRACK YOUR PROGRESS

TODAY

Weight	Measurements		How Do You Feel in Your Clothes?	What's Your Energy Level?
	Neck:	Waist:		
	Chest:	Hips:	1 2 3 4 5	1 2 3 4 5
	(L) Arm	(L) Thigh:		
	(R) Arm	(R) Thigh:		

Write down any negative thoughts, immediately cross them out, and replace them with a positive thought.

CANCEL-CANCEL BOX

. . . .

[PRO TIP] Stay neutral. Get curious!

. . . .

How Will You Conjure Up Additional Energy When Needed?

10 jumping jacks ___   Shout hypno-affirmations ___   Other ___

Water

8oz of water before breakfast ___   8oz of water before lunch ___   8oz of water before dinner ___

This Morning's Self-Hypnosis | Round 1: Week 11—Keep Going, Beat Resistance

Time you start: _____   Starting Stress Level (0–10): _____   Ending Stress Level (0–10): _____

This Afternoon's Self-Hypnosis | Round 2: Week 11—Keep Going, Beat Resistance

Time you start: _____   Starting Stress Level (0–10): _____   Ending Stress Level (0–10): _____

This Evening's Self-Hypnosis | Round 3: Week 11—Keep Going, Beat Resistance

Time you start: _____   Starting Stress Level (0–10): _____   Ending Stress Level (0–10): _____

Listen to this week's assigned hypnotherapy recording (found at www.CloseYourEyesLoseWeight.com): ☐

Tomorrow's Meal Planning

Breakfast	Snack	Lunch	Snack	Dinner

Check here when tomorrow's meals have been made or ordered: ☐

Visit www.CloseYourEyesLoseWeight.com and share your wins with our community: ☐

WEEK 11 LOG

DATE: __ / __ / __

TRACK YOUR PROGRESS

TODAY

Weight	Measurements		How Do You Feel in Your Clothes?	What's Your Energy Level?
	Neck:	Waist:		
	Chest:	Hips:	1 2 3 4 5	1 2 3 4 5
	(L) Arm	(L) Thigh:		
	(R) Arm	(R) Thigh:		

Write down any negative thoughts, immediately cross them out, and replace them with a positive thought.

CANCEL-CANCEL BOX

[PRO TIP] Stay neutral. Get curious!

How Will You Conjure Up Additional Energy When Needed?

10 jumping jacks ___   Shout hypno-affirmations ___   Other ___

Water

8oz of water before breakfast ___   8oz of water before lunch ___   8oz of water before dinner ___

This Morning's Self-Hypnosis | Round 1: Week 11–Keep Going, Beat Resistance

Time you start: _____   Starting Stress Level (0–10): _____   Ending Stress Level (0–10): _____

This Afternoon's Self-Hypnosis | Round 2: Week 11–Keep Going, Beat Resistance

Time you start: _____   Starting Stress Level (0–10): _____   Ending Stress Level (0–10): _____

This Evening's Self-Hypnosis | Round 3: Week 11–Keep Going, Beat Resistance

Time you start: _____   Starting Stress Level (0–10): _____   Ending Stress Level (0–10): _____

Listen to this week's assigned hypnotherapy recording (found at www.CloseYourEyesLoseWeight.com): ☐

Tomorrow's Meal Planning

Breakfast	Snack	Lunch	Snack	Dinner

Check here when tomorrow's meals have been made or ordered: ☐

Visit www.CloseYourEyesLoseWeight.com and share your wins with our community: ☐

WEEK 11 LOG

TRACK YOUR PROGRESS

TODAY

Weight	Measurements		How Do You Feel in Your Clothes?	What's Your Energy Level?
	Neck:	Waist:		
	Chest:	Hips:		
	(L) Arm	(L) Thigh:	1 2 3 4 5	1 2 3 4 5
	(R) Arm	(R) Thigh:		

Write down any negative thoughts, immediately cross them out, and replace them with a positive thought.

CANCEL-CANCEL BOX

- -

[PRO TIP] Stay neutral. Get curious!

- -

How Will You Conjure Up Additional Energy When Needed?

10 jumping jacks ___   Shout hypno-affirmations ___   Other ___

Water

8oz of water before breakfast ___   8oz of water before lunch ___   8oz of water before dinner ___

This Morning's Self-Hypnosis | Round 1: Week 11—Keep Going, Beat Resistance

Time you start: _____   Starting Stress Level (0–10): _____   Ending Stress Level (0–10): _____

This Afternoon's Self-Hypnosis | Round 2: Week 11—Keep Going, Beat Resistance

Time you start: _____   Starting Stress Level (0–10): _____   Ending Stress Level (0–10): _____

This Evening's Self-Hypnosis | Round 3: Week 11—Keep Going, Beat Resistance

Time you start: _____   Starting Stress Level (0–10): _____   Ending Stress Level (0–10): _____

Listen to this week's assigned hypnotherapy recording (found at www.CloseYourEyesLoseWeight.com): ☐

Tomorrow's Meal Planning

Breakfast	Snack	Lunch	Snack	Dinner

Check here when tomorrow's meals have been made or ordered: ☐

Visit www.CloseYourEyesLoseWeight.com and share your wins with our community: ☐

CHAPTER 15

· · · · · · · · · · · · ·

Week 12–
Learning to Love
Yourself for the
Long Run

Woohoo! You've reached the final week of our twelve-week program together. As you know, it's only the beginning of your lifelong journey to fall in love with your beautiful, magnificent body.

We started off with a brief discussion of self-love and are ending with it now. When you love your miraculous body right now, in this present moment, your choices will reflect the fact that you care about yourself.

Let's take a few moments to revel in the miracle that is your body.

Take a look at your nails. Look at how they grow. Isn't that incredible? Think about it.

Take a look at your knee. Look at how it bends and supports weight. Isn't that miraculous?

Move your toes around. Feel tremendous gratitude for how they move, how they help you balance, how wonderful those nubby little guys are. Say, "I love you, toes! Thank you for helping me walk."

Place your hands on your stomach and tell your tummy how sorry you are. "Stomach, I'm sorry, please forgive me, thank you, I love you. Thank you for digesting all my food, for being the place where my core strength emanates from, for putting up with all the negative things I've said to you and about you through the years. You are amazing. I'd be lost without you."

Look at your belly button, where you received nourishment in the womb. Think of how you were connected to your mother for nine months before you came into this world . . . Have you *ever* thanked your belly button for being a reminder of how freaking magical it is that you are alive?! Thank you, belly button!

Thank your ears for hearing the majesty that is music and children laughing.

Thank your head for growing hair.

Thank your eyes for seeing works of art, flowers, the ocean.

Thank your hands for typing and holding and creating.

Thank your lips for kissing.

Thank your spine and every single vertebra for helping you stand tall.

Thank your stretch marks for your gorgeous babies.

Thank your cellulite! Think of it like the rings of a tree that indicate its age, a new ring for every year. A beautiful marker for the passing of time. Of lived experience. Of wisdom.

Dimples? You are so cute! Wherever you are!

Thank your body. It's your only home.

Love your body. It loves you.

Cherish your body. It will notice.

Be kind to yourself.

Keep going.

You are worthy.

In this week's hypnosis recording and self-hypnosis practices, you will steep your subconscious in self-love and deep appreciation for your miraculous body.

Homework

A. Practice self-hypnosis three times a day, every day this week (right before breakfast, lunch, and dinner). Turn to page 20 for a reminder of how to do self-hypnosis or head to www.CloseYourEyesLoseWeight.com to follow along with a tutorial video.

Week 12 Hypno-affirmations—Self-Love

- I love you, heart. Thank you for beating.
- I love you, arms. Thank you for hugs.
- I love you, brain. Thank you for thinking.
- I love you, ears. Thank you for hearing.
- I love you, stomach. Thank you for turning helpful food into helpful fuel.
- I love myself, exactly as I am. I am perfect.

B. Listen to the "Week 12—Self-Love" hypnosis recording every day for the next week here: www.CloseYourEyesLoseWeight.com.

C. Use your journal pages daily to stay motivated, log your progress, and determine which pick-me-up hypno-affirmations you'll benefit from most.

WEEK 12 LOG

TRACK YOUR PROGRESS

TODAY

Weight	Measurements	How Do You Feel in Your Clothes?	What's Your Energy Level?
	Neck: Waist:		
	Chest: Hips:	1 2 3 4 5	1 2 3 4 5
	(L) Arm (L) Thigh:		
	(R) Arm (R) Thigh:		

Write down any negative thoughts, immediately cross them out, and replace them with a positive thought.

CANCEL-CANCEL BOX

[PRO TIP] Stay neutral. Get curious!

How Will You Conjure Up Additional Energy When Needed?

10 jumping jacks ___   Shout hypno-affirmations ___   Other ___

Water

8oz of water before breakfast ___   8oz of water before lunch ___   8oz of water before dinner ___

This Morning's Self-Hypnosis | Round 1: Week 12—Self-Love

Time you start: _____   Starting Stress Level (0–10): _____   Ending Stress Level (0–10): _____

This Afternoon's Self-Hypnosis | Round 2: Week 12—Self-Love

Time you start: _____   Starting Stress Level (0–10): _____   Ending Stress Level (0–10): _____

This Evening's Self-Hypnosis | Round 3: Week 12—Self-Love

Time you start: _____   Starting Stress Level (0–10): _____   Ending Stress Level (0–10): _____

Listen to this week's assigned hypnotherapy recording (found at www.CloseYourEyesLoseWeight.com): ☐

Tomorrow's Meal Planning

Breakfast	Snack	Lunch	Snack	Dinner

Check here when tomorrow's meals have been made or ordered: ☐

Visit www.CloseYourEyesLoseWeight.com and share your wins with our community: ☐

TRACK YOUR PROGRESS

TODAY

Weight	Measurements	How Do You Feel in Your Clothes?	What's Your Energy Level?
	Neck: Waist:		
	Chest: Hips:	1 2 3 4 5	1 2 3 4 5
	(L) Arm (L) Thigh:		
	(R) Arm (R) Thigh:		

Write down any negative thoughts, immediately cross them out, and replace them with a positive thought.

CANCEL-CANCEL BOX

[PRO TIP] Stay neutral. Get curious!

How Will You Conjure Up Additional Energy When Needed?

10 jumping jacks ___   Shout hypno-affirmations ___   Other ___

Water

8oz of water before breakfast ___   8oz of water before lunch ___   8oz of water before dinner ___

This Morning's Self-Hypnosis | Round 1: Week 12—Self-Love

Time you start: _____   Starting Stress Level (0–10): _____   Ending Stress Level (0–10): _____

This Afternoon's Self-Hypnosis | Round 2: Week 12—Self-Love

Time you start: _____   Starting Stress Level (0–10): _____   Ending Stress Level (0–10): _____

This Evening's Self-Hypnosis | Round 3: Week 12—Self-Love

Time you start: _____   Starting Stress Level (0–10): _____   Ending Stress Level (0–10): _____

Listen to this week's assigned hypnotherapy recording (found at www.CloseYourEyesLoseWeight.com): ☐

Tomorrow's Meal Planning

Breakfast	Snack	Lunch	Snack	Dinner

Check here when tomorrow's meals have been made or ordered: ☐

Visit www.CloseYourEyesLoseWeight.com and share your wins with our community: ☐

TRACK YOUR PROGRESS

TODAY

Weight	Measurements		How Do You Feel in Your Clothes?	What's Your Energy Level?
	Neck:	Waist:		
	Chest:	Hips:		
	(L) Arm	(L) Thigh:	1 2 3 4 5	1 2 3 4 5
	(R) Arm	(R) Thigh:		

Write down any negative thoughts, immediately cross them out, and replace them with a positive thought.

CANCEL-CANCEL BOX

[PRO TIP] Stay neutral. Get curious!

How Will You Conjure Up Additional Energy When Needed?

10 jumping jacks ___   Shout hypno-affirmations ___   Other ___

Water

8oz of water before breakfast ___   8oz of water before lunch ___   8oz of water before dinner ___

This Morning's Self-Hypnosis | Round 1: Week 12—Self-Love

Time you start: _____   Starting Stress Level (0–10): _____   Ending Stress Level (0–10): _____

This Afternoon's Self-Hypnosis | Round 2: Week 12—Self-Love

Time you start: _____   Starting Stress Level (0–10): _____   Ending Stress Level (0–10): _____

This Evening's Self-Hypnosis | Round 3: Week 12—Self-Love

Time you start: _____   Starting Stress Level (0–10): _____   Ending Stress Level (0–10): _____

Listen to this week's assigned hypnotherapy recording (found at www.CloseYourEyesLoseWeight.com): ☐

Tomorrow's Meal Planning

Breakfast	Snack	Lunch	Snack	Dinner

Check here when tomorrow's meals have been made or ordered: ☐

Visit www.CloseYourEyesLoseWeight.com and share your wins with our community: ☐

WEEK 12 LOG

TRACK YOUR PROGRESS

TODAY

Weight	Measurements	How Do You Feel in Your Clothes?	What's Your Energy Level?
	Neck: Waist:		
	Chest: Hips:	1 2 3 4 5	1 2 3 4 5
	(L) Arm (L) Thigh:		
	(R) Arm (R) Thigh:		

Write down any negative thoughts, immediately cross them out, and replace them with a positive thought.

CANCEL-CANCEL BOX

[PRO TIP] Stay neutral. Get curious!

How Will You Conjure Up Additional Energy When Needed?

10 jumping jacks ___   Shout hypno-affirmations ___   Other ___

Water

8oz of water before breakfast ___   8oz of water before lunch ___   8oz of water before dinner ___

This Morning's Self-Hypnosis | Round 1: Week 12–Self-Love

Time you start: _____   Starting Stress Level (0–10): _____   Ending Stress Level (0–10): _____

This Afternoon's Self-Hypnosis | Round 2: Week 12–Self-Love

Time you start: _____   Starting Stress Level (0–10): _____   Ending Stress Level (0–10): _____

This Evening's Self-Hypnosis | Round 3: Week 12–Self-Love

Time you start: _____   Starting Stress Level (0–10): _____   Ending Stress Level (0–10): _____

Listen to this week's assigned hypnotherapy recording (found at www.CloseYourEyesLoseWeight.com): ☐

Tomorrow's Meal Planning

Breakfast	Snack	Lunch	Snack	Dinner

Check here when tomorrow's meals have been made or ordered: ☐

Visit www.CloseYourEyesLoseWeight.com and share your wins with our community: ☐

WEEK 12 LOG

TRACK YOUR PROGRESS

TODAY

Weight	Measurements	How Do You Feel in Your Clothes?	What's Your Energy Level?
	Neck: Waist:		
	Chest: Hips:	1 2 3 4 5	1 2 3 4 5
	(L) Arm (L) Thigh:		
	(R) Arm (R) Thigh:		

Write down any negative thoughts, immediately cross them out, and replace them with a positive thought.

CANCEL-CANCEL BOX

[PRO TIP] Stay neutral. Get curious!

How Will You Conjure Up Additional Energy When Needed?

10 jumping jacks __   Shout hypno-affirmations __   Other __

Water

8oz of water before breakfast __   8oz of water before lunch __   8oz of water before dinner __

This Morning's Self-Hypnosis | Round 1: Week 12–Self-Love

Time you start: _____   Starting Stress Level (0–10): _____   Ending Stress Level (0–10): _____

This Afternoon's Self-Hypnosis | Round 2: Week 12–Self-Love

Time you start: _____   Starting Stress Level (0–10): _____   Ending Stress Level (0–10): _____

This Evening's Self-Hypnosis | Round 3: Week 12–Self-Love

Time you start: _____   Starting Stress Level (0–10): _____   Ending Stress Level (0–10): _____

Listen to this week's assigned hypnotherapy recording (found at www.CloseYourEyesLoseWeight.com): ☐

Tomorrow's Meal Planning

Breakfast	Snack	Lunch	Snack	Dinner

Check here when tomorrow's meals have been made or ordered: ☐

Visit www.CloseYourEyesLoseWeight.com and share your wins with our community: ☐

WEEK 12 LOG

TRACK YOUR PROGRESS

TODAY

Weight	Measurements	How Do You Feel in Your Clothes?	What's Your Energy Level?
	Neck: Waist:		
	Chest: Hips:	1 2 3 4 5	1 2 3 4 5
	(L) Arm (L) Thigh:		
	(R) Arm (R) Thigh:		

Write down any negative thoughts, immediately cross them out, and replace them with a positive thought.

CANCEL-CANCEL BOX

[PRO TIP] Stay neutral. Get curious!

How Will You Conjure Up Additional Energy When Needed?

10 jumping jacks ___   Shout hypno-affirmations ___   Other ___

Water

8oz of water before breakfast ___   8oz of water before lunch ___   8oz of water before dinner ___

This Morning's Self-Hypnosis | Round 1: Week 12—Self-Love

Time you start: _____   Starting Stress Level (0–10): _____   Ending Stress Level (0–10): _____

This Afternoon's Self-Hypnosis | Round 2: Week 12—Self-Love

Time you start: _____   Starting Stress Level (0–10): _____   Ending Stress Level (0–10): _____

This Evening's Self-Hypnosis | Round 3: Week 12—Self-Love

Time you start: _____   Starting Stress Level (0–10): _____   Ending Stress Level (0–10): _____

Listen to this week's assigned hypnotherapy recording (found at www.CloseYourEyesLoseWeight.com): ☐

Tomorrow's Meal Planning

Breakfast	Snack	Lunch	Snack	Dinner

Check here when tomorrow's meals have been made or ordered: ☐

Visit www.CloseYourEyesLoseWeight.com and share your wins with our community: ☐

WEEK 12 LOG

TRACK YOUR PROGRESS

TODAY

Weight	Measurements	How Do You Feel in Your Clothes?	What's Your Energy Level?
	Neck: Waist:		
	Chest: Hips:		
	(L) Arm (L) Thigh:	1 2 3 4 5	1 2 3 4 5
	(R) Arm (R) Thigh:		

Write down any negative thoughts, immediately cross them out, and replace them with a positive thought.

CANCEL-CANCEL BOX

[PRO TIP] Stay neutral. Get curious!

How Will You Conjure Up Additional Energy When Needed?

10 jumping jacks ___   Shout hypno-affirmations ___   Other ___

Water

8oz of water before breakfast ___   8oz of water before lunch ___   8oz of water before dinner ___

This Morning's Self-Hypnosis | Round 1: Week 12—Self-Love

Time you start: _____   Starting Stress Level (0–10): _____   Ending Stress Level (0–10): _____

This Afternoon's Self-Hypnosis | Round 2: Week 12—Self-Love

Time you start: _____   Starting Stress Level (0–10): _____   Ending Stress Level (0–10): _____

This Evening's Self-Hypnosis | Round 3: Week 12—Self-Love

Time you start: _____   Starting Stress Level (0–10): _____   Ending Stress Level (0–10): _____

Listen to this week's assigned hypnotherapy recording (found at www.CloseYourEyesLoseWeight.com): ☐

Tomorrow's Meal Planning

Breakfast	Snack	Lunch	Snack	Dinner

Check here when tomorrow's meals have been made or ordered: ☐

Visit www.CloseYourEyesLoseWeight.com and share your wins with our community: ☐

CHAPTER 16

· · · · · · · · · · · · · · · · · · · ·

You Did It! Now, How to Keep It Up?

You did it! You've made it to the end of this ninety-day cycle of rewiring your subconscious mind! Let's recap the major highlights of all you've learned:

- A distinction between what is "healthy" and what is *helpful* to your weight loss goals
- Solutions to the problems addictive foods create
- Stress relief (first prescriptive, then preventive by doing hypnosis four times per day)
- Realizing that, to lose weight, you must love the body you have now
- How to hypnotize yourself and how to write your own hypno-affirmations
- How to recognize and defeat Resistance
- The importance of chewing, hydrating, and stopping eating when you're 90 percent satisfied

- How to recognize and reframe subconscious limiting beliefs
- How to stop passing on wounding to the next generation
- How to trust your inner knowing more than any external rules or "favorite facts" and to eat intuitively (plus how blood tests can help)
- The importance of feeling your feelings and how to analyze them so emotional eating is stopped before it starts
- How to wake up from unconscious boredom eating
- How to use the law of attraction to expedite your weight loss goals by banishing any negative thinking toward yourself or your body
- How to stop "rewarding" yourself with poisonous punishments
- Strategies to avoid triggering people and places, plus what to do if there is a "slip-up"
- And so much more!

You've trained your brain to crave exercising. You've faced demons and have emerged strong with a deep conviction to live your bold, beautiful life. You've learned how to banish the yo-yo effect before it starts by anticipating the most likely times for Resistance to return. And finally, you've felt the rewards that come from thanking your body, your miraculous, beautiful body, for all it does, day in and day out.

By falling in love with the magnificence of who you are now, which includes your brilliant body, you are able to release weight in a natural, effective, noninvasive way that feels wonderful. Your body is a gift, it is your only home. Treat it with love, kindness, and respect by making helpful choices, all day, every day, and you will be rewarded with the body you desire.

Remember, hypnosis is a process of conditioning, albeit a quick one. If you've reached your weight loss goal in these past ninety days, wonderful! Keep chewing, keep drinking water, and switch up any hypno-affirmations that were focused on losing weight to make them about maintaining and staying right where you are. If you still have more pounds to go . . . rinse, wash, and repeat. Start from the top, keep tracking, keep going. You are worthy and deserving of seeing this through to the end. Make sure you visit www.CloseYourEyesLoseWeight.com to join our online community and find all the ways in which my team and I can support your success even further.

Thank you for taking the time to read what I've written for you. I'm honored you've dedicated so much of your precious time to being here with me. I'm proud of you. Keep it up! Be on the lookout for the next books in my Close Your Eyes series, which will help you with your sleep, stress, and more. Your mental freedom awaits. Until next time, tchau, tchau, beijos!

xx grace

P.S. Not ready to say goodbye yet? Me neither! Join me online for additional supportive resources at www.CloseYourEyesLoseWeight.com, including links to book private hypnotherapy sessions, to enroll in my hypnotherapy certification school, to download our app, and so much more!

Acknowledgments

My heartfelt thanks go out to so many; this book would not be here without you! To my dear husband and partner in everything, Bernardo, for being my rock. Patrick, my beautiful son, thank you for being an endless source of inspiration for me. To my parents, Joni and George, for their unconditional love and support.

To my literary agent, Lisa Gallagher, for believing in me when my "office" was the size of a closet in Union Square, NYC, and every step of the way since.

To Joshua Lisec for all of your wonderful coaching and ongoing support.

To everyone at BenBella (Adrienne Lang, Sarah Avinger, Alicia Kania, Susan Welte, Lindsay Marshall, Monica Lowry, and the many others who worked on this book behind the scenes!) for all of your hard work and for making this book series a reality. Special thanks to Glenn Yeffeth for welcoming me into the BenBella family and to Vy Tran for countless hours of editing and support!

To all of our Grace Space Hypnosis team members, clients, customers, students, and friends for your ongoing love and support and for being committed to making the world a better place through your own subconscious healing.

To our backstage pass members who provided such wonderful questions, feedback, and support throughout the writing of this manuscript, thank you! Backstage pass members: Marise C., Lisa S., Lauren M., Nancy F., Ginni G., Kira P., Kristine A., Karen B., Julie K., Wendy S., Tony O., Julian M., Amie R., Dena D., Paul K., Wendy D., Trish M., Jourdan R., Jenna B., Jacqueline M., Kathy B., Marianne K., Stephanie D., Holly C., Renee B., Linda M., Darlene M., Riki S., Tracy C., Aida R., Angel W., Anna K., Wendy C., Joselyn A. V., Elizabeth E., Sarah K., Kelly H., Valerie B., Anjanette F., Elizabeth R., Barbara P., Catherine G., Catherine K., Vicki P., Art R., Angela P., Maria R., Shannon M., Dina U., Stephanie R., Colleen R. D., Laura H., Jean L., Annette L., Eva A., Kristin R., Jamie H., Carol R., Brooke B., Leesa S., Denise R., Julie E., Meegan S., Lisa M. H., Sandra W., Teresa K., Adrian A., Lexi T., Meike H., Helene A., Trish G., Beth H., Angela M., Santa L., Amy C., Claire M., Margi H., Christian A., Betty S., Joan F., Tammy A., Laura C., Nadine E., Ta H., Katherine G., David H., Lindsay V. N., Alexis D., Linda S., Christina I., Alicia A., Maritza D., Susanne H., Kristin M., Stefanie L., Joy B., Carly V., Angela T., Lewis C., Danie M., KK M., Megan F., Anu R., Gretchen B.

It takes a massive village to publish a book. I'm infinitely grateful to everyone mentioned, as well as all of my dear friends and family who helped me navigate the highs and lows of authorship so this book could become a reality. Thank you, thank you, thank you.

With love,
grace

About the Author

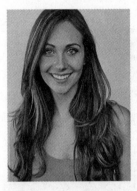

Grace Smith is on a mission to make hypnosis mainstream. As a pioneer in the hypnotherapy field, her private clients include Fortune 500 CEOs, celebrities, and government officials.

Grace is the founder of Grace Space Hypnosis, the world's number one provider of hypnosis education, products, and services (visit www.gshypnosis.com),

Photo by Mikaela Gauer

and Grace Space Hypnotherapy School, a world-class hypnotherapy certification program (visit www.gshypnosis.com/school).

Grace is the author of the number one Amazon best seller *Close Your Eyes, Get Free: Use Self-Hypnosis to Reduce Stress, Quit Bad Habits, and Achieve Greater Relaxation and Focus*.

Her work has been featured on *The Dr. Oz Show*, in the *Atlantic*, *Forbes*, *Entrepreneur*, *InStyle*, *Marie Claire*, BuzzFeed, Bustle, mindbodygreen, SheKnows, and dozens of podcasts. She is a regular guest on CBS's hit show *The Doctors*, and her Relax, Brazil! segment on the popular Brazilian late-night talk show *The Noite com Danilo Gentili* brought her powerful self-hypnosis technique into the homes of millions of viewers.

Grace's keynote speeches include OZY Fest with Hillary Clinton, the international Women's Leadership Academy, FEMConnect with Procter & Gamble, SummitLive, Women Empowerment Expo, Soul Camp, and more.

To learn more about Grace, follow her on Instagram @gracesmithtv. To work with Grace as a private client or hire her to speak at your next event, visit www.gracesmithtv.com.

For all other hypnosis products and services, including worldwide private hypnotherapy phone sessions with graduates of Grace Space Hypnotherapy School, visit www.gshypnosis.com.

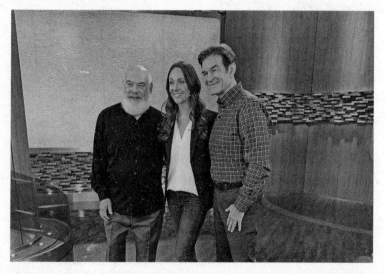

Grace on *The Dr. Oz Show* with Dr. Andrew Weil to discuss hypnotherapy for pain relief (as a safe, noninvasive alternative to opiates and surgery).